M000014795

Living with Lung Cancer

A GUIDE FOR PATIENTS AND THEIR FAMILIES

Second Edition

Barbara G. Cox, M.A., Ed.S.
and
David T. Carr, M.D.

Robert E. Lee, M.D.
Contributor

Illustrations by John W. Desley

TRIAD PUBLISHING COMPANY GAINESVILLE, FLORIDA

Copyright 1987 by Barbara G. Cox and David T. Carr

All rights reserved. No part of this book may be reproduced in any manner without written permission of the publisher.

Printed in the United States of America

Published and distributed by
Triad Publishing Company, Inc.
1110 Northwest Eighth Avenue
Gainesville, Florida 32601

Library of Congress Cataloging-in-Publication Data

Cox, Barbara G.
Living with lung cancer.

Includes index.
1. Lungs--Cancer--Popular works. I. Carr, David T.
II. Lee, Robert E., 1926- . III. Title.
(DNLM: 1. Lung Neoplasms--popular works. WF 658 C878L)
RC280.L8C69 1987 616.99'424 86-25655
ISBN 0-937404-19-5 (pbk.)

For information on bulk orders write: Special Sales Dept., Triad Publishing Company, 1110 N.W. 8th Avenue, Gainesville, FL 32601.

To the patients and families
whose collaboration made this
book possible.

The National Cancer Institute, National Institutes of Health, funded preparation of the first edition of *Living with Lung Cancer* and its revision for the second edition.

Contents

Foreword

From the First Edition

The key to the more successful approaches to controlling and curing cancer is the basic message of this book—teamwork. A physician in the past had little knowledge and few adequate tools, other than the surgeon's scalpel, to combat cancer, and he was "on his own." Today, comprehensive cancer centers are demonstrating that the best, most successful way to control cancer is to combine the knowledge and skill of numerous medical specialists to plan and execute the best treatment for each patient. Cancer is a complex disease and requires complex and integrated means to control it.

And, along with the new medical philosophies of good cancer care must develop new attitudes on the part of cancer patients. No longer is it appropriate for a patient to assume a passive role in treatment, to be someone the physicians "do something to." Each patient is and should be a very active member of the cancer team. Patients' attitudes and behavior during the course of therapy are essential elements in the potential success of the treatment.

This book is an invitation to you to understand and to join the team to help yourself.

R. LEE CLARK, M.D.
PRESIDENT
THE UNIVERSITY OF TEXAS
SYSTEM CANCER CENTER

Preface

At long last, we are converting the black box that once was the cancer cell into a blueprint of the growth and development of living organisms. The technology of the biologic revolution has allowed us to peer inside the cell and begin to track the genes involved with cell growth and the switches that turn them on and off. Whereas in the past this kind of information usually was first appreciated and applied in practice to cancers less common than those derived from the lung, the new biology now applies to all cancer cells, and lung cancer is no exception. Genes that go awry and lead to uncontrolled growth (oncogenes) have been identified in lung cancer and, in some cases, the products of these genes have been identified and used as targets for the newest treatment programs. This is just the tip of the iceberg of things to come.

What does all this mean to the patient with lung cancer? In this book, the multidisciplinary team approach to the management of the disease is emphasized. This team has been saddled with treatments difficult to administer and with limited effectiveness, although many patients owe their lives to the effectiveness of this approach. With the new biology upon us treatments will now have to face a new, equally challenging, if somewhat more pleasant problem, the orderly integration of this steady stream of new information, and the practical tools that result, into the day-to-day care of the patients with lung cancer. This type of work has never been easy. The practical application of new knowledge for every disease requires the judicious mixing of the new with the old, to avoid prematurely abandoning tried and true methods, and it requires overcoming logistical difficulties, socioeconomic problems, and yes, sometimes even the habits and resistance of traditional medicine.

However bleak an individual case may seem, the best chance a patient has of capitalizing on this new knowledge is a thorough understanding of the disease and the assurance of care by such a team of health providers that has the required experience and is also enthusiastic about the prospects of developing new approaches that will eventually overcome lung cancer. This book describes the former and outlines the important elements of the latter.

VINCENT T. DEVITA, JR., M.D.
DIRECTOR, NATIONAL CANCER INSTITUTE
BETHESDA, MARYLAND

Introduction

This book was written to help patients live with lung cancer. And to help their families live with them. We believe that knowledge is strength and that knowledge about lung cancer will enable patients and their families to understand their problems and to face them with courage and patience.

This is not an encyclopedia. We have not included everything that is known about lung cancer. However, we have attempted to tell the truth about lung cancer, giving many of the unpleasant facts about the disease but emphasizing that much can be done to help the patient and sometimes even cure the cancer. The subjects in the book range from a brief history of lung cancer to current research that promises to yield better ways to treat this disease. The book has been written so that it can be kept on the shelf as a ready reference source, or so that it can be read from cover to cover.

The idea for the book and its title came from one of the authors (D.T.C.), a physician who has specialized in the treatment of patients with lung cancer for many years. Dr. Carr's patients have repeatedly requested reading materials about lung cancer, but until now nothing appropriate was available, There were only lengthy, highly technical descriptions in the medical textbooks or a scattering of popular books about cancer that were far too general for most patients.

Because writing a book in lay language that would answer all the questions patients and their families had about lung cancer promised to be a huge task, Dr. Carr enlisted the aid of two colleagues. He also applied for and received financial support for the project from the National Cancer institute. His colleagues in the project were Ms. Barbara G. Cox, a medical writer whose specialty is patient education and cancer rehabilitation, and Dr. Robert E. Lee, a radiotherapist whose specialty is the treatment of lung cancer patients.

The project began with tape-recorded interviews of lung cancer patients and their spouses. Ms. Cox and an associate spent countless hours interviewing these individuals to determine what they wanted to know about lung cancer, and particularly what they thought should be included in this book. The transcripts of these interviews formed the starting point for the book manuscript.

Months of tape-recorded interviews of health professionals followed, with Drs. Carr and Lee providing Ms. Cox with the bulk of technical information for the book. But many others contributed, too—surgeons. radiotherapists, medical oncologists, nutritionists, and social workers. Medical textbooks were reviewed, as well. When Ms. Cox had compiled information from all these sources and had written the first draft of the book, it was submitted for critical review to twenty physicians who were experts in the treatment of lung cancer. They made many helpful suggestions.

Finally, a draft of the book was ready for patient evaluation. This was the acid test. Patients with lung cancer and their families acted as the final arbiters of what should be in the book. These individuals—over twenty in all—graciously agreed to be our "editors." They reviewed the book manuscript in detail. They filled out questionnaires about the content of the book, penciled in their suggested revisions directly on the manuscript pages, and, finally, were interviewed at length by Ms. Cox. These tape-recorded sessions were later transcribed.

During Ms. Cox's interviews with these patients and their families, they revealed that they had countless questions about lung cancer that were often difficult to ask in a doctor's office. They said that they badly needed background information to help them cope with the disease, its treatment, and, perhaps most of all, their nameless fears about lung cancer. Many patients and families had canvassed the bookstores in search of information, but everything they found was too general. Others confessed that they had resorted to medical dictionaries and textbooks in the public library without telling their doctors, only to come away more confused than ever. This book, *Living with Lung Cancer*, was exactly what they needed, they told us.

This is not to say that they glossed over the book without criticism. The patients and family members who reviewed the book were tough, honest "editors." They made important recommendations on the questionnaires we gave them, changed the manuscript in a number of places, and, in their interviews with Ms. Cox, told us what they thought should be added to the book. (This introduction is an example.) They even suggested illustrations that they thought would be helpful to readers. The drawings that they suggested are oversimplified in many cases, especially the anatomical drawings—but this was done to make our basic ideas clear to lay readers.

The information in the pages that follow was edited by patients for patients. They knew how desperately they had wanted information about lung cancer, and they gave long hours of their time so that others might be more well informed. They also reinforced our belief that patients and their families need to share information in order to cope with the problems that accompany lung cancer. To the people who helped us write this book, knowledge was a weapon against lung cancer—a weapon they wanted us to pass on to you.

Living with Lung Cancer

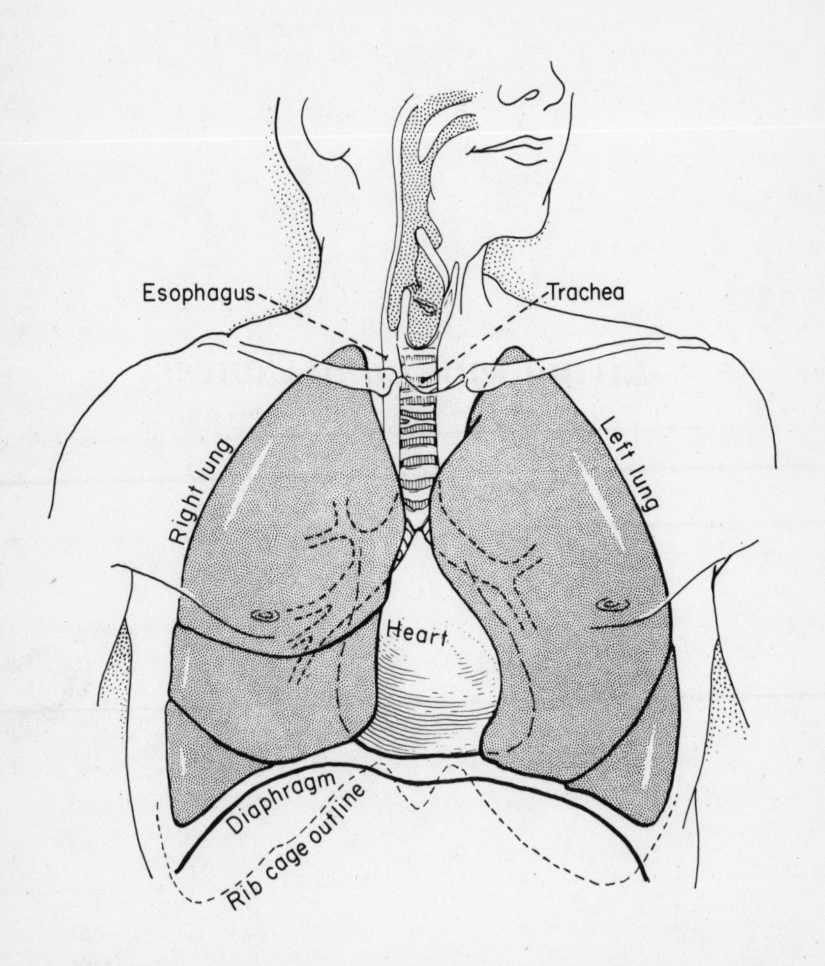

The chest, showing the trachea (the windpipe), its division into the right main bronchus and left main bronchus, and the lungs on each side. The esophagus (the swallowing tube) is beside the trachea, and the heart is between the two lungs. The diaphragm, which forms the floor of the chest, is below the lungs and the heart.

CHAPTER 1

The Lungs and How They Work

The lungs are two spongy, pinkish-gray organs that make up the major part of your breathing apparatus. They extend from high in the chest, just above the collarbones, to the bottom of the rib cage.

Each lung is made up of sections called *lobes*. The right lung is slightly larger than the left and has three lobes. The left lung has two lobes. It is smaller because the heart takes up part of the space on the left side of the chest.

The left lung folds around the heart, and both lungs fold around the large blood vessels and the *esophagus* (the tube that carries food from the mouth to the stomach). All the organs in your chest are contained inside the rib cage, which surrounds and protects them. At the bottom of the rib cage, making a sort of floor for the lungs, is the *diaphragm*, a sheet of muscle that helps you draw air into the lungs when you breathe.

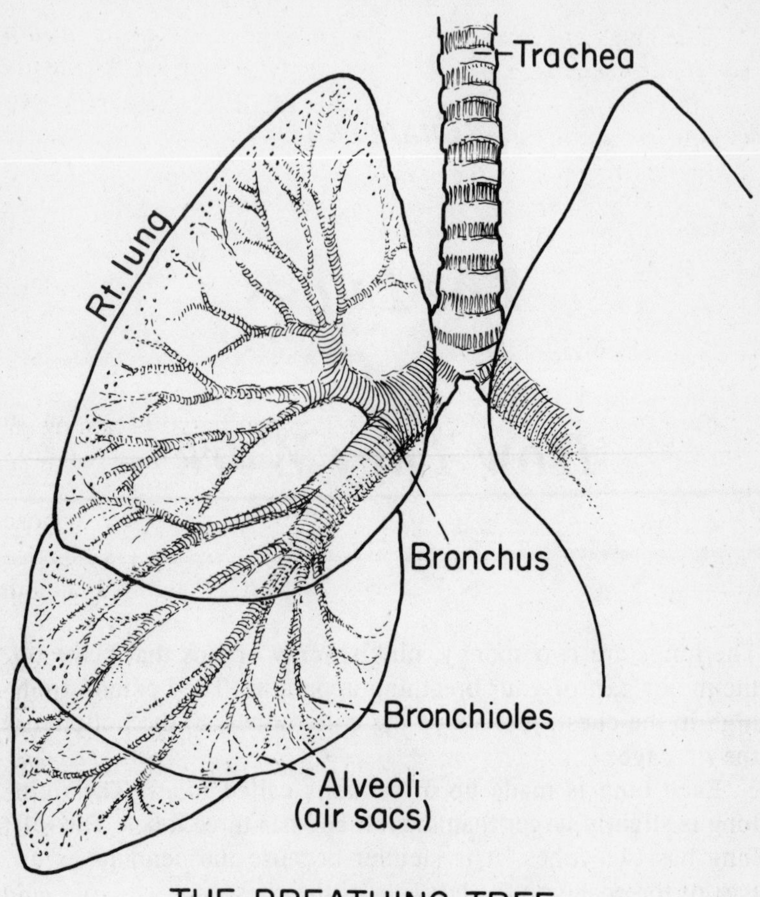

THE BREATHING TREE

The "breathing tree," showing the trachea and its division into the right main bronchus and left main bronchus. The right main bronchus is shown dividing into branches that enter the lobes of the right lung, where they subdivide into smaller and smaller branches. The smallest branches, the bronchioles, connect to the alveoli (the air sacs).The left lung contains the same structures.

The lungs are covered by a thin membrane called the *pleura* (or *pleural membrane*). A similar membrane lines the inside of the chest cavity. A thin layer of fluid separates these two membranes, lubricating them so they can slide on each other when you breathe. In a similar way, tears lubricate your eyes and the inside surface of your eyelids.

What Happens When You Breathe

Respiration (breathing) consists of two parts: breathing in (also called inhalation or inspiration) and breathing out (exhalation or expiration).

The air you breathe is inhaled through your mouth or nose and eventually reaches the lungs. Along the way, the air passes through a system of tubes that resemble the trunk, limbs, and branches of an upside-down tree.

Air first enters the *larynx* (voicebox). From there it flows through the main breathing tube, the *trachea* (windpipe); in the illustration this is the "trunk" of the tree. The trachea goes down the neck into the chest, where it branches into two *bronchi*. One bronchus leads to the right lung and the other leads to the left. The trachea and bronchi are held rigid and open by stiff rings of cartilage around the outside of the tubes.

Inside each lung the bronchus divides into smaller and smaller branches and then into *bronchioles*, tiny tubes that are almost too small to see. These carry the air to all parts of the lung. At the far end of each bronchiole is a cluster of tiny air sacs (called *aveoli*). Each air sac is surrounded by the smallest blood vessels of the body—each thinner than a thread—which are called *capillaries*.

Each lung contains hundreds of millions of alveoli (air sacs), and it is here that the work of the lung really goes on.

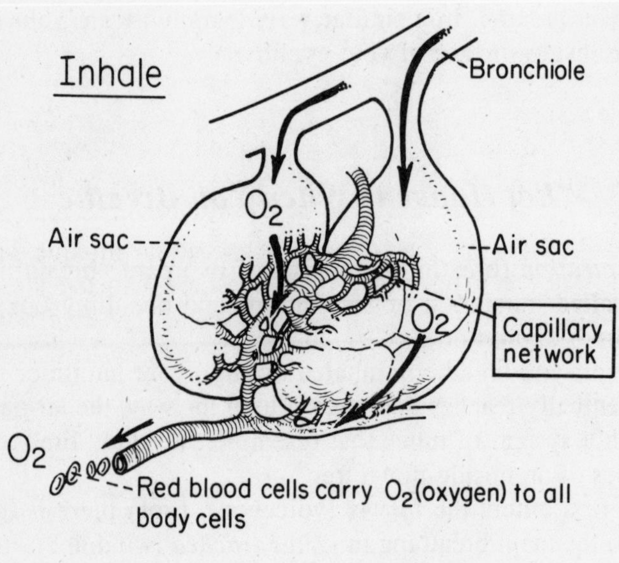
Inhale
Bronchiole
O_2
Air sac
Air sac
O_2
Capillary network
O_2
Red blood cells carry O_2(oxygen) to all body cells

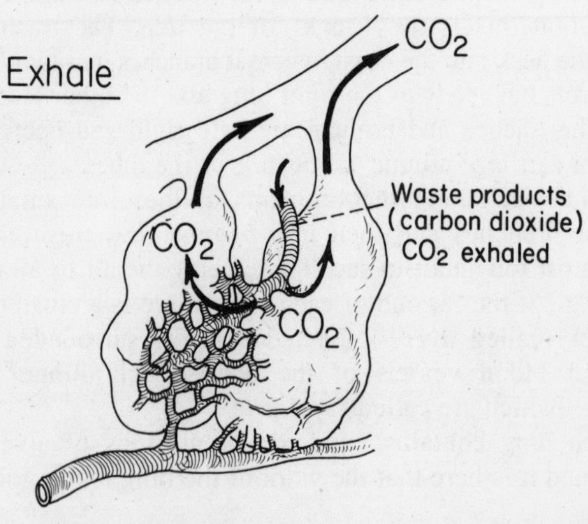
CO_2
Exhale
Waste products (carbon dioxide) CO_2 exhaled
CO_2
CO_2

The oxygen-rich air you have breathed in passes into the air sacs. From there the oxygen passes through a thin membrane and enters the tiny blood vessels, where it is carried by red blood cells to the heart. The heart then pumps blood containing oxygen to all the cells in the body. This function of heart and lungs together is necessary for life, since the cells of the body need oxygen to stay alive.

The body cells that take in oxygen must also get rid of carbon dioxide, a waste product. So the process reverses. The cells return carbon dioxide to the bloodstream, to be carried back to the heart. The heart pumps the blood and carbon dioxide back to the lungs, where the carbon dioxide passes from the tiny blood vessels (the capillaries) to the air sacs. The air containing carbon dioxide then travels from the smaller to the larger branches of the "breathing tree" and, as you breathe out, leaves your body.

Inhalation *(top)*. A tiny bronchiole connected to two alveoli (air sacs) during inhalation. The capillary network (only part of which is shown) covers the alveoli. The oxygen in the air that enters the alveoli during inhalation passes through the wall of the alveoli into the blood flowing through the network of capillaries.

Exhalation *(bottom)*. As oxygen passes from inhaled air into the alveoli and from the alveoli into the blood in the capillary network, carbon dioxide (CO_2) passes from the blood into the alveoli. The carbon dioxide is then exhaled through the bronchioles into the larger bronchial tubes, on into the trachea, and out through the mouth or nose.

How the Lungs Work

Consider how a bellows works to fan a fire. When a bellows expands, air is sucked in. When it is compressed, air is blown out. The diaphragm and the other muscles in the chest work together with the elastic tissue in the lungs to make your lungs expand and contract. Like the bellows, as you breathe in the lungs expand, drawing in oxygen-rich air. As you breathe out the lungs contract, forcing out waste carbon dioxide.

The breathing process is under the control of a "breathing center" in your brain. The brain coordinates the entire breathing cycle, so that each part in the cycle works at the proper time and in the proper way. That is what makes the rib cage muscles and diaphragm expand and contract as you breathe in and out.

CHAPTER 2

How Lung Cancer Begins

Lung cancer is the uncontrolled growth of abnormal cells in the lung. Most lung cancers begin on the moist inner lining of one of the breathing tubes. This is why you may hear lung cancer also called *bronchogenic carcinoma, bronchial carcinoma*, or *cancer of the bronchus*.

Normal Cells

Cells are the microscopic units that make up every part of our bodies. There are many different kinds of cells, and there is a tendency for each kind to be specific in appearance and specialized in what it does. Normal cells grow in an orderly, controlled pattern. As they wear out and die, new ones are produced to replace them.

Several kinds of cells line the breathing tubes. One type of cell produces the thin layer of mucus that covers the inner surfaces. The mucus traps foreign particles, such as dust, from the air that flows in and out of the lungs. Other cells have tiny hairs, called *cilia*, that continually sweep this

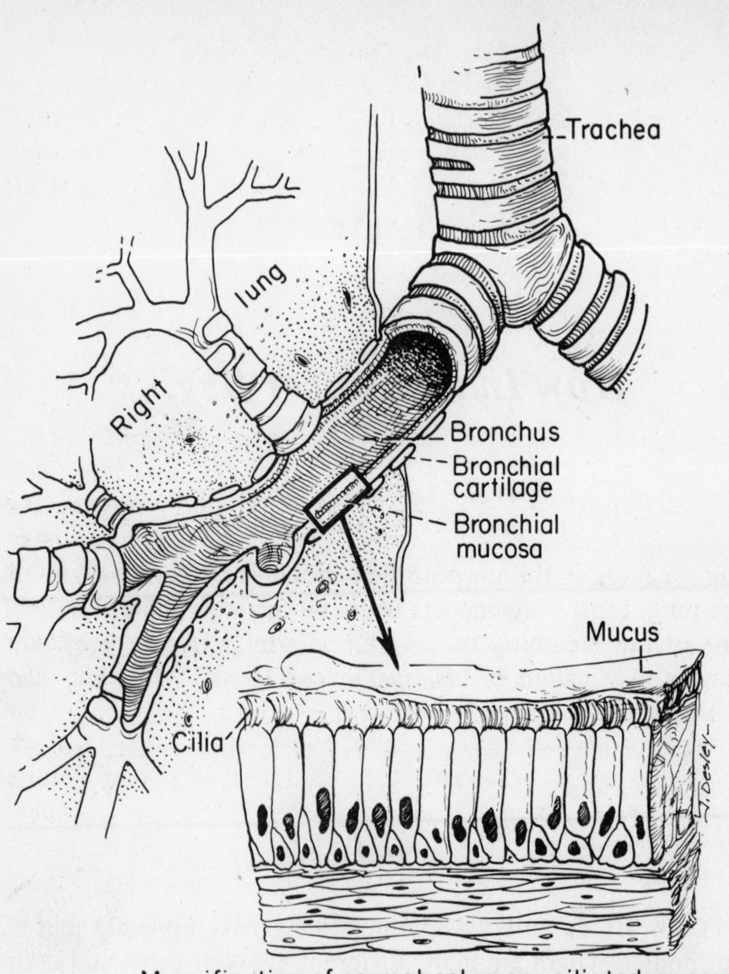

The trachea and right main bronchus and its divisions. Part of the wall of the bronchus is cut away to show the layers of the wall and the film of mucus that covers the inside of the bronchus. The inset shows a magnification of the wall with the tall columnar cells arising from the basal cells. The columnar cells have hairlike projections, called cilia, that sweep back and forth to move the mucus upward into larger and larger bronchi, into the trachea, and up into the throat to be swallowed. By catching dust particles that enter the "breathing tree" with the inhaled air, the mucus protects the delicate air sacs.

mucus upward toward the throat and out of the body. Both of these kinds of cells help cleanse the lungs of foreign substances such as particles of tobacco smoke and other air pollutants.

How Normal Cells Become Cancerous

Cancer (also called *carcinoma*) develops when normal cells change, become abnormal, and grow in an uncontrolled manner. Scientists are still not certain what triggers the change from normal cells to cancer cells. While we have learned a great deal about this in recent years, a number of the pieces of the puzzle are still missing.

Scientists think that lung cancer develops very slowly from a "precancerous" condition in which the cells lining the breathing tubes become damaged by dirty air, especially air containing tobacco smoke. Most cancer researchers believe that twenty or more years pass from the time a person starts inhaling a cancer-producing substance, such as tobacco smoke, and the time cancer actually develops.

Unfortunately, we still have no reliable tests to detect precancerous cells in the lungs. However, microscopic studies of the sputum and lung tissue of heavy smokers show that, during this precancerous period, some of the cells start to look different from those around them. Once this happens, we do not know how to reverse the process.

At some point, however, the damaged cells may stop growing in orderly rows, like normal cells do, and begin to grow in abnormal arrangements. Eventually, the abnormally arranged cells change into outright cancer cells. The cancer cells destroy normal cells and replace them with more cancer

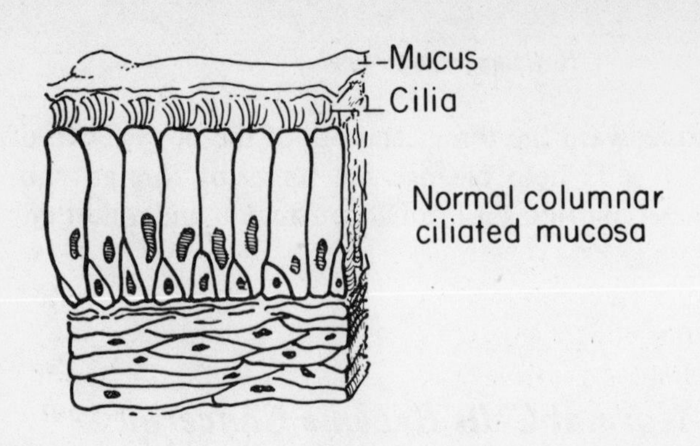

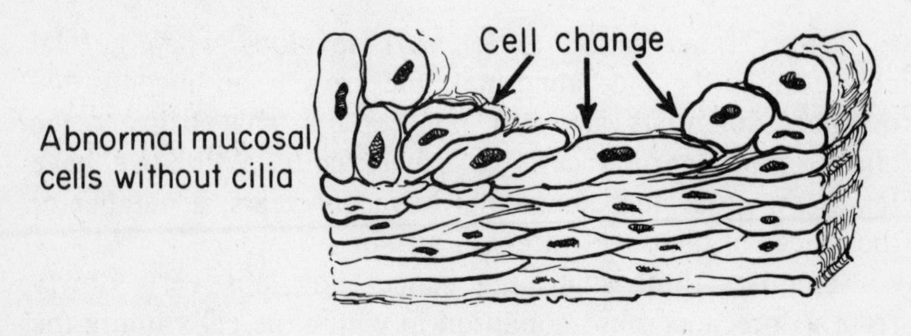

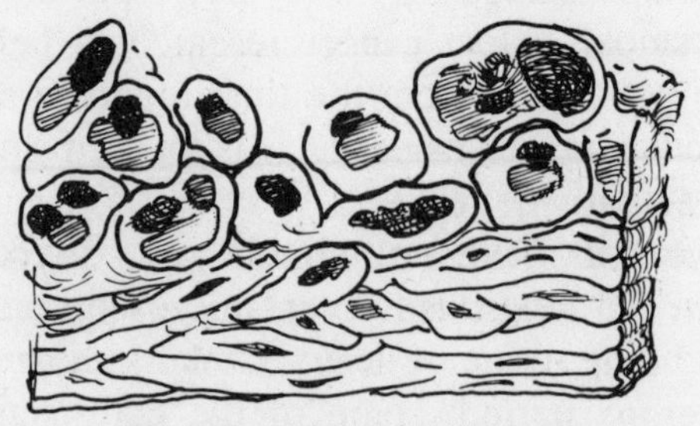

Magnified sections of the wall of a bronchus showing the changes from normal tissue to the beginning of a cancer. *Top*: Normal bronchial mucosa is made of up of the basal cells, the columnar ciliated cells, and the blanket of mucus. *Middle*: Abnormal bronchial mucosa lacks the columnar ciliated cells and the layer of mucus. *Bottom*: The abnormal cells have deteriorated further into cancer cells. This is the beginning of a cancer of the bronchus.

cells. From then on, all future generations of these cells are cancerous.

One characteristic of abnormal cells in the breathing tubes is that they lack the tiny hairs, or cilia. When this happens, the mucus secretion can no longer be swept upward and out of the breathing tubes. Instead, you may find it necessary to raise the mucus that collects in the breathing tubes by coughing it up and spitting it out. Sometimes you may cough it up and swallow it.

Cancer cells grow and multiply without regard for the healthy functioning of the organs in the body. In the lungs or breathing tubes, the cells that once helped the breathing process are replaced by cancer cells that do not serve this function.

How Fast Does Lung Cancer Grow?

From the time of the first abnormal cell changes, every type of cancer grows at its own specific rate, different from other forms of cancer. (Surprisingly, even cancer obeys some rules.) Lung cancer is one of the slowly growing tumors. In its earliest stages, doctors cannot detect it on X-ray pictures. Then, when the tumor is large enough to be diagnosed, it may be hard to cure.

A tiny clump of cancer cells may take three to four months to double in size. Many patients, not aware of how slowly the cancer grows and frightened by their diagnosis, feel they need to rush ahead with tests and treatment. They've probably heard that lung cancer is an emergency. It is not, and a few days' delay is not dangerous.

Doubling Time

Doctors use the term "doubling time" in predicting how fast a tumor will grow. Doubling time is the time required for the cells to reproduce themselves one time, meaning that the tumor will double in size. Many lung cancer cells take three to four months to double. A single cell would require about thirty doubling times for the tumor to become one-half inch (1 centimeter) in diameter, the size at which it can first be detected on a chest X-ray. (One cell would become two cells, then four, then eight, sixteen, thirty-two, etc.) A one-half inch tumor would contain about one billion cells.

To calculate how long it would take for a one-half inch tumor to develop from one cancerous cell, multiply 30 (the number of doubling times to reach that size) by 3 (the number of months the cell needs to double one time). Thirty times 3 equals 90 months. This means that about seven and a half years are needed for that first cancer cell to double and redouble enough times to make a half-inch tumor.

How Fast Should You Act?

As you can see, lung cancer is a chronic disease. Therefore there is no need to panic and feel that something must be done immediately. Your tumor has probably grown to its present size over a period of years, and a difference of a few days won't make a great deal of difference.

Your doctors know when action must be taken rapidly and when tests and treatments can be planned and carried out in a more deliberate, less hurried way. They will plan a diagnosis and treatment schedule that works best for you.

How Lung Cancer Spreads to Other Parts of the Body

A malignant tumor in one part of the body can spread to other locations in the body. This happens when cells break away from the original tumor and travel through the body via the bloodstream or lymphatic system. This process is often called "seeding."

Metastases

When a tumor that has been "seeded" by the lung cancer starts to grow in another part of the body, such as the liver or a bone, we call it a *metastasis*. The new growth is not a different kind of cancer, such as "liver cancer" or "bone cancer." It is simply lung cancer that has moved into distant territory and begun to grow there. It is called "metastatic lung cancer." Because of metastases, the first symptoms of lung cancer sometimes occur in a totally different part of the body.

Metastases keep at least some of the characteristics of the original tumor, so doctors may treat them in the same way as they treated the original tumor. For example, if a lung tumor responds well to chemotherapy, the treatment is also likely to be effective against metastases from that tumor.

Some people wonder why a metastatic tumor sometimes grows to be larger than the original tumor. Lung cancers consist of a mixture of cancer cells, some that grow rapidly and some that grow slowly. If the cancer cells that escape from the lung are the rapidly growing type, they may grow into a larger tumor than the primary one in the lung.

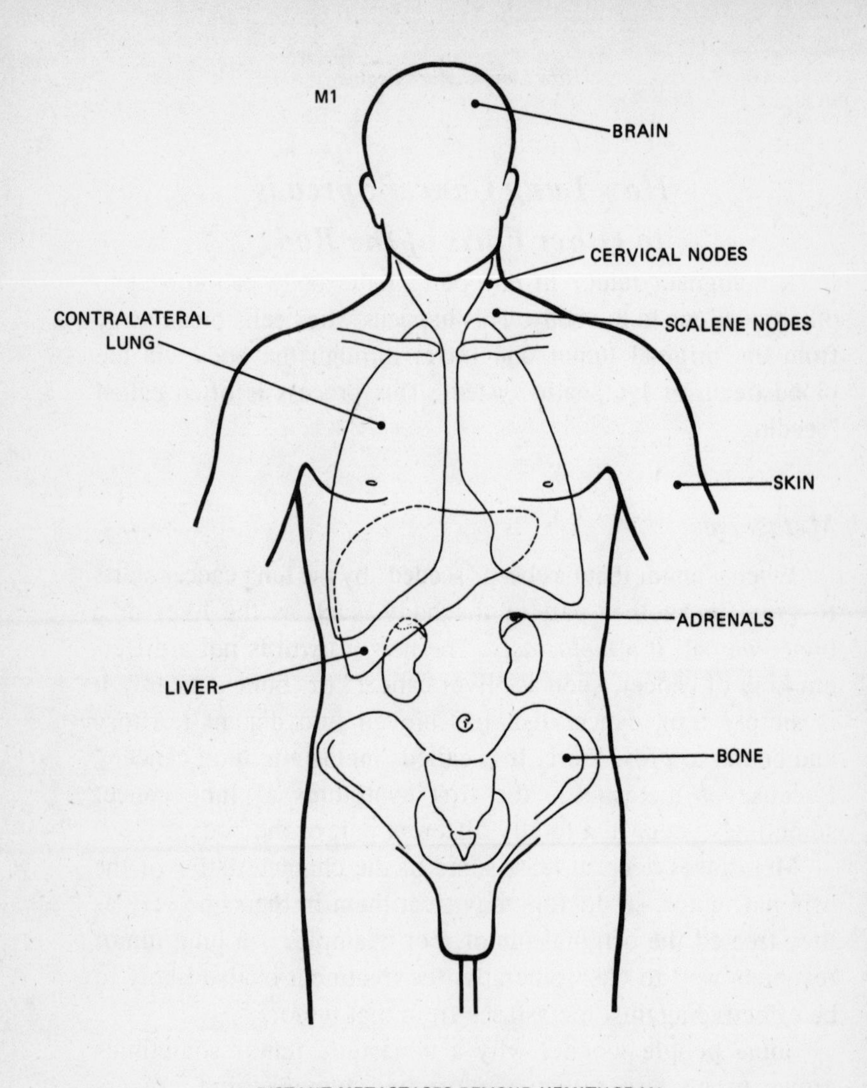

DISTANT METASTASES BEYOND HEMITHORAX

The organs in the body to which lung cancer spreads most frequently. When the cancer has spread to an organ outside the lung, it is called a metastasis. Sometimes the metastasis causes symptoms and is diagnosed before the tumor in the lung is detected.

The Lymphatic System

Your body has a network of lymph vessels that resembles its network of blood vessels. The purpose of the lymph vessels is to drain *lymph*, a clear fluid, from the body tissues. The lungs, too, have a system of lymph vessels that drain lymph from lung tissues.

Throughout the body, lymph is absorbed by the smallest lymph vessels, which carry it into larger and larger lymph vessels. Finally, the fluid is emptied into veins in the neck where it mixes with the blood. Along the branches of the lymph vessels lie *lymph nodes*, clusters of bean-shaped nodes that trap germs and other microscopic foreign objects, like cancer cells. In this way, lymph nodes act to slow down or stop the spread of disease.

Cancer cells traveling through the lymphatic system may become trapped in the lymph nodes and multiply there. That is why many patients with lung cancer have enlarged lymph nodes filled with cancer cells. Actually, the body's natural defense mechanisms are trying to stop the cancer from spreading. However, some cells escape from the nodes, to plant themselves and grow in other parts of the body.

Even though lung cancer grows slowly, it can spread throughout the body faster than most other tumors because the lungs have such a rich supply of blood and lymph vessels. Lung cancer probably spreads more slowly through the lymphatic system than through the bloodstream because the lymph nodes act as temporary traps for cancer cells.

How a Tumor May Affect Your Lungs and Other Organs

For a long time, a lung tumor may be only a small spot of cancer cells on the lining of a breathing tube and may not affect the rest of the lung at all. As it grows, it may block the free flow of air through the breathing tube, resulting in a wheeze or a whistling noise. A growing tumor may also interfere with the normal movement of mucus up and out of the lungs, causing a cough or making an existing cough worse. If the tumor blocks a main breathing tube, it can cause shortness of breath. If the breathing tube is blocked badly enough, the mucus made in the bronchial tubes can't be swept upward past the tumor and out of the lungs, as it normally would. So it collects in the lung, causing a type of pneumonia.

Sometimes small ulcers appear on a lung tumor, making it bleed. You may see streaks of blood in the mucus that you cough up. Heavy bleeding, however, is rare. If the tumor spreads to the outside surface of the lung, it may cause fluid to collect in the pleural cavity, the space between the lung and ribs. The symptoms are chest pain and difficulty in breathing.

Sometimes a tumor spreads directly from the lung into the tissues of the chest wall, causing pain. Or it may grow from the lung toward the center of the chest, between the lungs, and press on the esophagus (swallowing tube). This pressure may make swallowing difficult until the tumor is found and treated.

If a lung tumor presses on the blood vessels that carry blood to and from the heart, the normal blood flow may be blocked. In some patients, the tumor may damage one of the nerves that go to the larynx (voice box), causing hoarseness.

Sometimes cancer cells start to grow in one of the bronchioles (the smallest branches of the breathing tree) near the aveoli (the tiny air sacs). Here, the tumor can become the size of a golf ball or even larger without causing symptoms. Although the tumor can be seen on a chest X-ray picture, the patient may not be aware of its presence for years.

Causes of Lung Cancer

Patients often ask, "What causes lung cancer?" Scientific research indicates that smoking is the major cause, but it is by no means the only one.

A small proportion of lung cancer patients have never smoked but have lung cancer due to other causes. For example, exposure to asbestos and other substances can produce lung cancer. Miners who work with certain radioactive ores have often been victims of the disease. Researchers have found that the incidence of lung cancer is higher among city-dwellers than among people who live in the country, suggesting that pollution in the city air plays an important role.

One thing is certain. People who have been exposed for many years to irritating substances in the air, including secondhand smoke, are more likely to have lung cancer than people who have breathed unpolluted air all their lives. So far, tobacco smoke has proven to be the main villain.

Researchers also believe that the tendency to get lung cancer may be inherited. Clinical studies suggest that blood relatives of lung cancer patients are more apt to get the disease than people who have no such family history.

Since all heavy smokers don't get lung cancer, those smokers who do must be especially sensitive to the effects of tobacco smoke. The same seems to be true for people who are heavily exposed to all the other air pollutants and chemicals that may cause lung cancer.

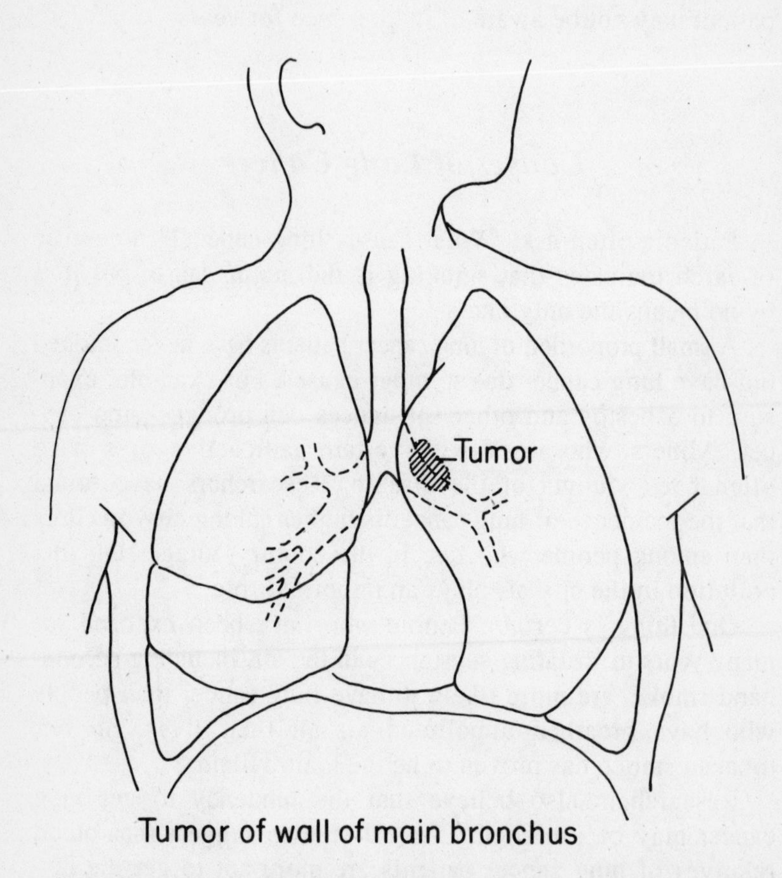

Tumor of wall of main bronchus

A tumor of the left main bronchus that partially obstructs it. Breathing through the narrowed bronchial tube sometimes produces a wheezing noise. Growth of the tumor could block the bronchus completely and cause shortness of breath. Retention of mucus beyond the tumor might cause pneumonia in the affected lung. If the tumor ulcerates, it might cause bleeding and coughing up of bloody sputum.

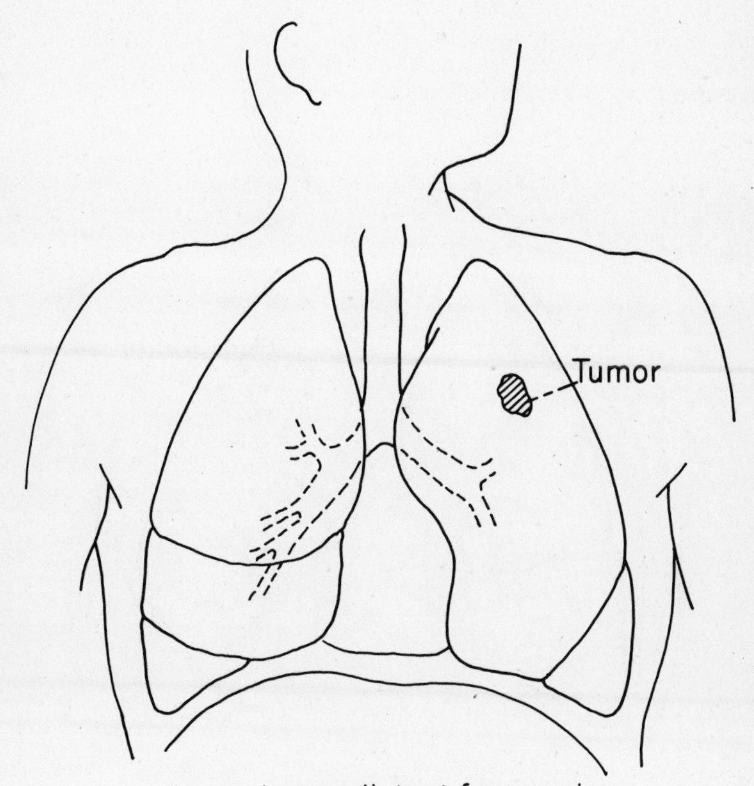

Small tumor distant from main bronchus

A small tumor in the upper part of the left lung. This type of tumor often starts in one of the small bronchial tubes and causes no symptoms. It can be detected on a routine chest X-ray film. Surgical removal of such a tumor frequently cures the patient.

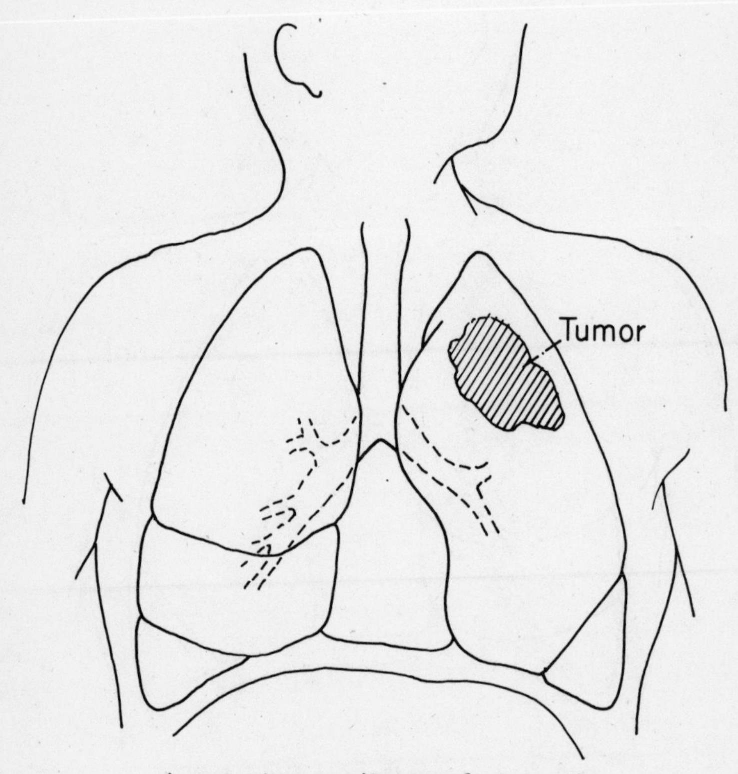

Large tumor distant from main bronchus

A large tumor in the upper part of the left lung. Such a tumor can grow for several years and cause no symptoms. It can be detected easily by a routine chest X-ray film. Surgical removal is possible and may cure the patient.

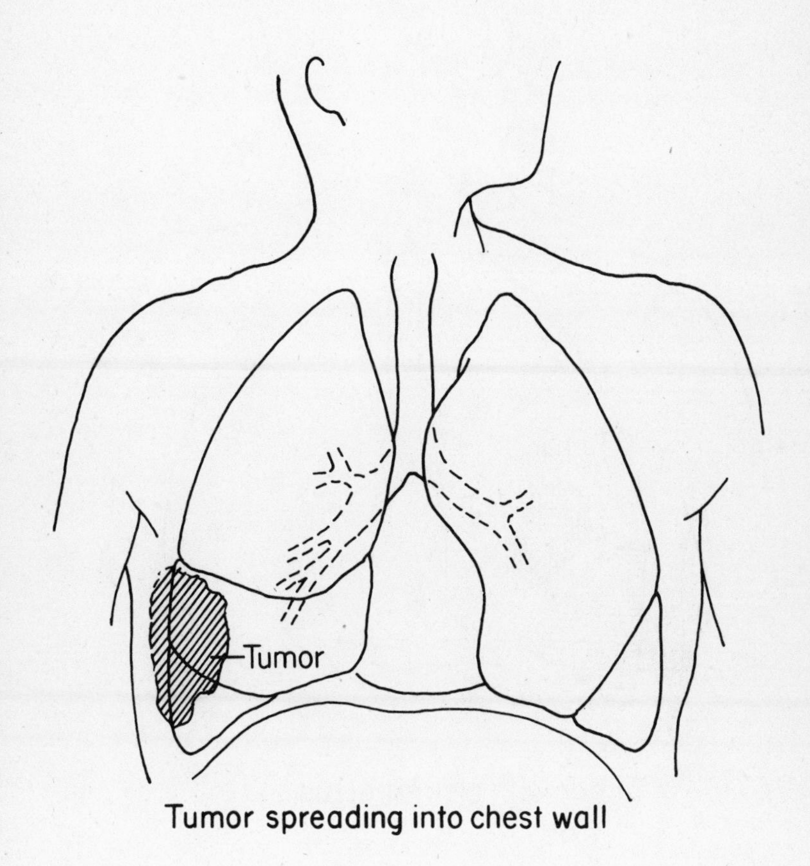

Tumor spreading into chest wall

A large tumor in the right lung that has grown directly from the lung into the chest wall. This type of tumor often causes pain in that part of the chest. Such tumors can sometimes be removed surgically along with the involved chest wall, completely curing the patient.

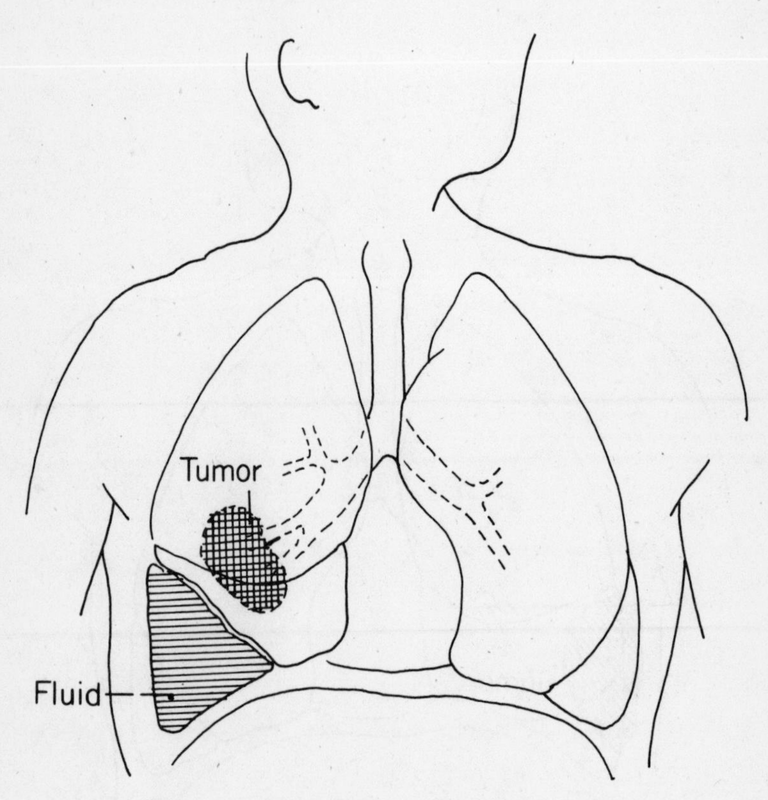

Tumor with pleural effusion...

A large tumor in the right lung that has caused fluid to collect in the space between the lung and the ribs. This type of fluid collection, called a "pleural effusion," sometimes causes pain in the chest. The amount of fluid can increase, fill up the right side of the chest, and completely collapse the lung, causing shortness of breath.

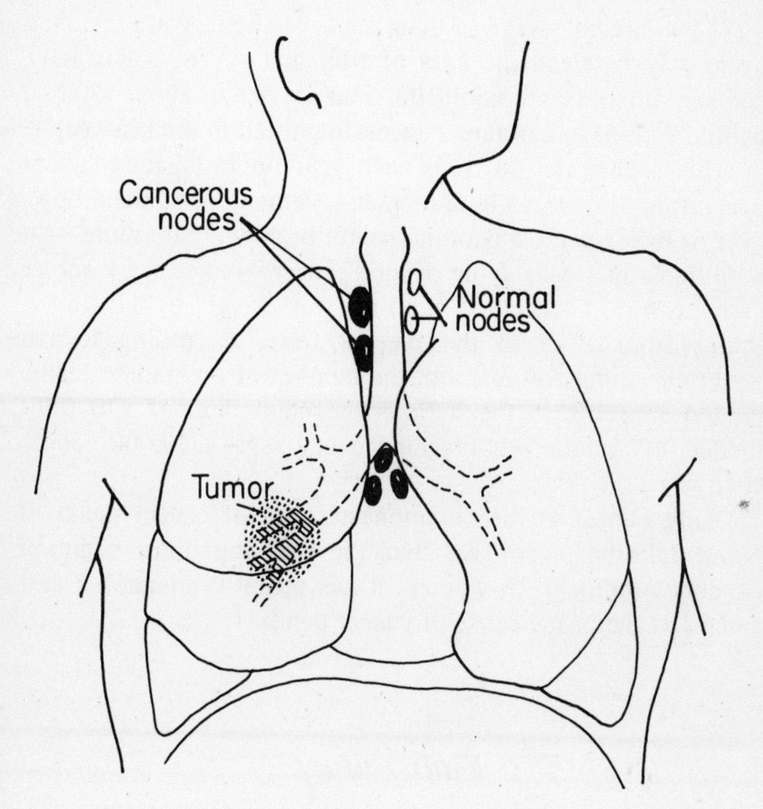

Tumor with metastases to mediastinal nodes

A tumor in the right lung with spread to the lymph nodes in the mediastinum between the two lungs. Such tumors are usually treated with radiotherapy and chemotherapy only. Surgical removal of such a tumor is sometimes possible but usually does not cure the patient, so radiotherapy and/or chemotherapy are often given after the operation.

Who Gets Lung Cancer?

If you are an "average" lung cancer patient, you are a man or woman between the ages of fifty and seventy. You have smoked most of your adult life. You are one of about 150,000 people who have had lung cancer diagnosed in the last year.

This "epidemic" worsens each year. In 1930, lung cancer was a rare disease, in both men and women. Since then, however, it has become a national health problem, with more than a million Americans dying of lung cancer—more than twice as many as have been killed in all the wars fought by the United States from 1775 to the present time. According to the American Lung Association, the number of premature deaths due to smoking in the U.S. is the equivalent of 920 fully loaded 747 jumbo jets crashing every year—350,000 people each year.

Lung cancer is the commonest cause of cancer death in men, claiming more lives than the next four most common cancers combined. In women, it has recently replaced breast cancer as the prime cause of cancer death.

Your Future

If your lung cancer is diagnosed in its early stages, the chances of cure are good. Many patients who have a lung tumor removed surgically stay well for five years and more after the operation. Even if your cancer has spread outside the lung, modern treatment may enable you to you may live a comfortable, productive life for a long time after the diagnosis.

CHAPTER 3

How Lung Cancer Is Diagnosed

For some patients, lung cancer is discovered during a routine annual check-up, usually when it is found on a chest X-ray. In general, though, patients develop symptoms that prompt them to see a doctor.

Symptoms

Many patients see the doctor when a long-term cigarette cough gets worse. Or, more commonly, they become alarmed by blood in their sputum. About half of the people with lung cancer cough up mucus with flecks or streaks of blood. Some patients have fever and yellow or green sputum as the first symptoms; these can occur when the cancer plugs one of the breathing tubes. Chest pain is another common symptom.

Sometimes the first symptoms occur in a different part of the body because of a metastasis from the original tumor. A patient might have headaches or dizziness from a metastatic tumor in the brain. Another might have bone pain, caused by a metastatic tumor in the bone.

What the Doctor Looks For

A doctor who suspects lung cancer needs to find out first if you really have lung cancer, or whether your symptoms are the result of some other lung problem. The doctor can gain valuable information about your condition by taking a health history and giving you a physical examination and diagnostic tests.

Your health history offers clues to the diagnosis. For example, if you are a long-time smoker who has recently started coughing up blood, lung cancer will be suspected as the cause. The physical examination is also important. A hard lump in the neck, for example, suggests that a cancer may have spread from some nearby part of the body to the lymph nodes in the neck.

If your physical examination and initial tests suggest that you do have lung cancer, your doctor then needs to find out where the tumor is and how big it is before planning your treatment. If it seems likely that the tumor is confined to a small area in the lung, surgery will probably be performed in an attempt to remove all the cancer and thereby cure you. If, on the other hand, tests indicate that the disease has spread to other parts of the body, treatment must be aimed at stopping or slowing the growth of the cancer cells in these areas.

Diagnostic Tests

Many different kinds of tests may be used to determine whether or not you have lung cancer. There are several kinds of X-ray examinations and your doctor will decide which ones you need. Other methods of obtaining a picture of the inside of the body have been developed, and these will be used if needed. The sputum, blood, urine, and other body fluids will be examined. Instruments may be used to look into various parts of the body, and in some cases specimens will be taken for examination in the laboratory. If necessary, an operation may be performed to complete the diagnosis.

Although some people believe that lung cancer can be diagnosed by a blood test, this is not true. Blood tests may help determine whether the cancer has spread to an organ such as the liver, but such tests must be done in conjunction with other studies.

Once the diagnosis of lung cancer is certain, other questions must be answered, such as, has the cancer spread beyond the lung? If so, where and to what extent? Also, what type do you have?

The most commonly used tests are described below.

Chest X-Ray

Since lung cancer can usually be seen on the X-ray film as an abnormal shadow, a chest X-ray is one of the first tests you will have. As with most types of X-ray pictures, this test causes no discomfort.

The smallest tumor that can be seen on a chest X-ray is about one-half inch in diameter (a little over 1 centimeter). But even if the tumor itself is not seen, the chest X-ray may offer other clues to the diagnosis of lung cancer. One such clue is pneumonia in the lung. Another is enlarged lymph nodes (which may be filled with cancer cells). A third is pleural effusion, an accumulation of fluid in the space between the lung and the chest wall. Lung cancer is not always the cause of these, but they are signs that alert the doctor to look for the cause, using other diagnostic tools.

Sometimes the doctor will want you to have a chest X-ray even if the diagnosis is already clear. The purpose is to be able to compare it with previous and later X-rays, to follow your progress and watch for possible changes in the lung tissue. It is important for your doctor to find out whether the cancer is growing, or whether it is responding to treatment and shrinking.

Tomogram

A tomogram is a series of X-ray pictures of various sections of lung tissue. When put together, they give a three-dimensional image of any abnormal shadow. Like a regular X-ray, a tomogram will cause you no discomfort.

If a regular chest X-ray has shown a suspicious shadow in the lung, a tomogram may reveal more about the size, shape, and characteristics of the tumor. Sometimes a tomogram will reveal enough about a tumor that the doctor can tell that it is not cancer. If it does suggest that a tumor is malignant, however, additional studies will be needed to be sure of the diagnosis.

CAT Scan

A CAT scan, or CT scan, is a recently developed type of tomogram that can create a three-dimensional image from any area of the body. (CAT stands for computerized axial tomography.) This is a valuable diagnostic tool that combines

X-rays, an electronic information-gathering system, and a computer. As with other types of X-ray tests, a CAT scan involves no discomfort. The only thing that tells you that scanning is taking place is a soft whirring noise.

In the test, the X-ray portion of the equipment moves back and forth, scanning all the dimensions of an area in which a tumor is supected. It can pick up images of tumors that are too small to be detected by other kinds of X-rays. It may also be able to detect areas of spread before troublesome symptoms have a chance to start. If you already have a diagnosis of lung cancer, your doctor may want you to have a CAT scan of the brain or of the organs in your chest or abdomen, the most frequent areas of spread.

Specialized X-Rays

There are several other kinds of specialized X-ray studies. One is the *bronchogram*, which is a picture of the breathing tubes. This X-ray is made after some liquid has been injected into the breathing tubes, which allows them to show clearly on the film. The injection of the fluid may be uncomfortable, but a local anesthetic is used to reduce the discomfort. In some cases X-rays may be made while the patient lies down or after all the air has been exhaled.

Ultrasound

Ultrasound is a relatively new technique in which high-pitched sound waves (that the human ear cannot hear) are sent into your body. The sound waves are bounced back by the body structures and picked up by a converter that changes them into a picture called a *sonogram*. This, too, is a painless examination.

The sonogram is particularly useful for examining the abdominal organs for spread of cancer and for detecting collections of fluid around the heart or between the lungs and the ribs.

MRI (Magnetic Resonance Imaging)

MRI (formerly called nuclear magnetic resonance) is an experimental diagnostic method that resembles X-ray techniques, but does not expose the patient to X-rays. The process involves the use of a huge magnet to align the protons of the body cells in such a way that pictures of the various internal organs can be obtained. MRI is valuable because it can be used to take pictures of any part of the body. Again, there is no discomfort.

The equipment is large, expensive, and must be housed in a special room or even a separate building. For these reasons, most community hospitals may be unable to experiment with or develop MRI for practical use. So far, we do not know if it will prove to be a valuable addition to the X-ray examinations now in use, or whether it will replace one or more of them.

Sputum Cytology

"Cytology" means the study of cells, and sputum cytology means, simply, the examination of a sample of your sputum under a microscope for signs of cancer cells. If cancer cells are present, the type of cells may also be determined.

Different doctors may use slightly different methods of sputum collection. You may be asked to cough up some mucus (or sputum) and spit it into a bottle. Or you may be given a bottle containing a preservative and asked to collect specimens of your sputum over a period of several days or at specific intervals.

If you should have a cluster of cancer cells in the breathing tubes, some of these cells are likely to be shed and carried up to your throat in the sputum. After the sputum is collected, it will be placed on glass slides to be studied under a microscope.

If you are not coughing very much and cannot easily raise sputum by making yourself cough, you may be asked to inhale a warmed mist that stimulates your breathing tubes to produce more mucus than usual. This mist also causes you to cough.

Bronchoscopy

Bronchoscopy is a technique that enables the doctor to look directly into your breathing tubes. The instrument that makes this possible is called a *fiberoptic bronchoscope.*

The bronchoscope is made up of tightly packed, long glass fibers that transmit a light into the breathing tubes and carry a "picture" back to the examiner's eye. It can go around corners as it passes through your nose, throat, and breathing tubes.

The doctor will spray a local anesthetic into your throat and breathing tubes to make them numb, so that you are not too uncomfortable during the procedure. The bronchoscope will be inserted into only one breathing tube, so you will have no trouble breathing. In addition, the doctors and nurses will watch your breathing and pulse carefully to be sure that your heart and lungs continue to function normally throughout the examination.

If a tumor is seen, a cutting instrument can be passed through the bronchoscope, to snip out a small sample of tissue. This tissue is then studied under a microscope to find out if it contains cancer and, if so, what kind. Samples of mucus and other secretions will also be taken for examination in the laboratory.

You may cough up a small amount of blood after the examination. This frequently happens and should be no cause for alarm.

Biopsy

Biopsy means obtaining a small piece of tissue and examining it with a microscope. A biopsy specimen may be removed from your lungs during bronchoscopy or during any one of several surgical procedures done for diagnosis, for treatment, or for both. If lung cancer has spread to the lymph nodes in the neck or to other body tissues, a specimen of these might be taken for biopsy. In some cases, a needle may be used to aspirate material to be examined for cancer cells.

The pathologist studying the biopsy tissue can usually identify the cell type of the lung cancer along with its degree of malignancy. Findings from the biopsy examination are important in determining what treatment plan is best for you.

Mediastinoscopy

Mediastinoscopy is a minor operation. It is done to find whether lung cancer has spread to the chain of lymph nodes behind the breastbone, one of the first places lung cancer is likely to spread.

A small incision is made in the middle of the neck, through which a long, slender instrument is passed down behind the breastbone area. If you have this operation, you will be anesthetized and asleep while it is being done. Lymph nodes will be removed and sent to the pathologist's laboratory for examination. The decision to proceed with further surgery will depend upon several considerations, including what cell type the cancer is and your general condition. Often a thoracotomy is done after the mediastinoscopy to gain more information about the operability of your tumor.

Thoracentesis

Thoracentesis is a procedure in which a needle is used to remove fluid from the space between the lungs and chest wall. The fluid is studied with a microscope for the presence, and type, of cancer cells. Thoracentesis is usually done when other attempts at finding cancer cells have failed. Sometimes it is done to relieve pain or shortness of breath caused by the collection of fluid in the pleural space.

The procedure can take place in a hospital room or an examining room. To minimize discomfort, a local anesthetic is applied to the skin before the needle is inserted. Gentle suction will draw the fluid through the needle into a syringe or a bottle. Sometimes a biopsy of the pleural membrane is performed also.

Thoracoscopy

Thoracoscopy is a relatively new surgical procedure for diagnosing lung cancer. It is used when fluid has collected between the lungs and the chest wall, and/or when examination of the fluid does not show cancer cells. If you have this operation, you may be anesthesized and asleep in the operating room.

A small incision is made between two ribs, through which a *thoracoscope* is inserted. A thoracoscope is a long, slender instrument much like the fiberoptic bronchoscope. The instrument is flexible, so it can be used to examine almost the entire surface of the lung for tumor growth. The lining of the chest wall can also be searched for signs of cancer. If tissue is found that looks malignant, a small piece is snipped off, withdrawn through the thoracoscope, and sent to the pathologist for microscopic examination.

Thoracotomy

Thoracotomy is a diagnostic procedure that is done when all other tests have failed to locate the tumor or clarify its nature or extent. It is a major operation in which the surgeon opens up one side of the chest enough to examine the lung. It is performed in the operating room with the patient anesthetized and asleep.

An incision is made between two ribs, extending from the shoulder blade in back around to the front just under the nipple. Part of a rib may be removed. The ribs are spread apart enough for the surgeon to be able to see inside. While one lung is worked on, the other lung continues to breathe. The heart and lungs are both monitored during the entire operation to be sure they are functioning properly.

This operation allows careful and complete exploration of the lung. It is done when the doctor is reasonably sure that lung cancer is present and that there is a chance of cure. If a tumor is found, a specimen may be removed and sent to the laboratory. The pathologist examines the tissue with a microscope and sends the report to the operating room within minutes.

If the pathologist's report indicates that the cell type of the tumor is favorable for operation, and the surgeon finds no evidence of metastases (disease spread), the lung or a part of it is usually removed. In this way, both the diagnosis and the surgical treatment are done during one operation.

Other Procedures

Most of the remaining diagnostic procedures are for finding out whether the cancer has spread to any other organs. For example, if you have pain that feels as if it comes from bone, the doctor will probably arrange for you to have a test called a bone scan. A bone scan is painless, much like an X-ray.

Before the scan is done, a small amount of sterile, radioactive liquid is injected into a vein in your arm. The amount of radioactivity is small and is harmless to you. If there are any cancerous spots in the bone, they will absorb the radioactive liquid and show up on the bone scan, alerting the doctor that the disease has probably spread to that bone. The doctor will then check for metastatic cancer with X-rays of those bones.

The liver is another place where lung cancer cells can start growing. Your doctor may order a liver scan if your liver feels abnormally large during the examination. A liver scan is also done if certain blood tests indicate that the liver is not working properly.

Types of Lung Cancer

Many patients are surprised to learn that there are more than a dozen different kinds of lung cancer. The type of cells found in the tumor determines the kind. The identification of cell type is made by a pathologist, who examines a sample of tumor tissue, and possibly mucus from your lung, sputum, and/or pleural fluid under a microscope.

How your lung cancer is treated and how successful your treatment is depends partly on the cell type. For example, small epidermoid carcinomas and adenocarcinomas (described below) can be cured by an operation in a large percentage of patients. Other types of cancer are more difficult to cure, although modern treatment methods can often bring them under control for long periods of time.

The following four types are the most common, making up more than ninety percent of all cases of lung cancer:

Epidermoid carcinoma. This type of tumor (also called *squamous cell carcinoma*) usually starts in one the larger breathing tubes and grows relatively slowly. There may be great variability in size at the time of diagnosis.

Small cell carcinoma. This type of tumor (also called *oat cell carcinoma*) usually starts in one the larger breathing tubes, grows fairly rapidly, and is likely to be large by the time of diagnosis.

Adenocarcinoma. This type starts growing near the outside surface of the lung and may vary in both size and growth rate. Some slowly growing adenocarcinomas are called *alveolar cell cancer*.

Large cell carcinoma. This type starts near the surface of the lung, grows rapidly, and is usually large when diagnosed.

The names of some of the uncommon types of lung cancers are *carcinoid, cylindroma, mucoepidermoid*, and *malignant mesothelioma*.

Malignant mesothelioma is of special interest because more patients have been found to have it in recent years. A mesothelioma is not a cancer of the lung itself, but develops on the pleural membrane lining the chest cavity or, less often, on the pleural membrane covering the lung. However, its symptoms and the way doctors diagnose and treat it are similar to lung cancer.

Malignant mesothelioma is usually caused by the inhalation of asbestos fibers. Many people have worked with asbestos and inhaled some of the fibers into their lungs. Others have been exposed because city air has been polluted with asbestos fibers from the construction or demolition of buildings and from the wearing away of automobile brake linings, which are usually made of asbestos.

Once the asbestos fibers get into the lungs, they remain there permanently; apparently, the irritation of the pleural membrane by the fibers causes some people to get malignant mesothelioma. During and after World War II, asbestos use increased greatly, accounting for the increase in the number of patients getting malignant mesothelioma. Fortunately, the use of asbestos is now being controlled, so the number of patients with this type of malignancy should decrease in the future.

Classifications of Lung Cancer

Some types of lung cancer are also classified by the degree of malignancy. They are identified as Grades I, II, III, and IV. Grade I is the least malignant; it grows most slowly and is least likely to spread. Grade IV is the most malignant. Grades II and III are, of course, in between.

Most hospitals also use a "staging" system, called the TNM classification, which gives doctors an accurate picture of the extent of the disease and the chances for cure. TNM numbers are assigned to a cancer to give doctors specific information about its size and location.

The T number refers to how big the tumor is. A tumor of about one inch in size (3 centimeters or less) is classified as T1. A T2 is larger.

N describes the degree of lymph node involvement. N0 means that no nodal involvement can be seen, and N1 means that only certain lymph nodes in the lung or near it contain cancer.

The M number tells the extent of metastases outside the chest. M0 means that no distant metastases have been found, and M1 means that the doctors have found a metastasis in an organ such as the liver.

In TNM staging, a T1 N0 M0 lung cancer means that the original (primary) tumor is not more than three centimeters across, that the lymph nodes in or right next to the lung do not contain cancer, and that no lung cancer cells have been found in other parts of the body. This is called Stage 1 lung cancer and is the most curable of the four stages. Stages 2, 3 and 4 are more advanced but also may be curable. How your cancer needs to be treated is related to its stage as well as the cell type.

Improving Patients' Lives

If you have lung cancer, its treatment depends on complete diagnostic findings. Your doctor can order the diagnostic tests needed to determine whether your cancer can or cannot be cured, and then develop an effective treatment plan for you.

As you shall see in the chapters that follow, the treatment of lung cancer has improved in recent years. Often the life span of patients is lengthened considerably by surgery, radiotherapy, chemotherapy, or a combination of these.

If the cancer cannot be cured, there may be treatments that will slow or stop the tumor's growth for periods of time. The complete diagnosis of the extent of disease also allows your doctor to prescribe treatment that will keep you as comfortable as possible and will minimize symptoms. Much depends on your type of lung cancer and its stage.

Modern medical care now assures a patient relief from most of the cancer's troubling symptoms. Patients can enjoy a much more comfortable life than they could in years past. Although some patients find that they need to cut down their activities somewhat, many keep on working and enjoy an active social life as well. In fact, patients often stress the importance of carrying on a normal life and not giving up the pleasures of work and leisure.

CASE REPORT: ROBERT DAWSON*

Robert Dawson is an accountant who smoked two packs of cigarettes a day for many years.

After his graduation from high school during World War II, he tried to enlist in the army. When he was rejected (because of handicaps remaining from an attack of polio in childhood), he went to work in a shipyard, building Liberty ships. During this time, he worked with asbestos without knowing that it was dangerous material. Many of his co-workers smoked cigarettes so he learned to smoke along with them, never realizing that this, too, was harmful to his health. No one knew then that the combination of asbestos and tobacco smoke was so deadly.

After the war he went to college to study accounting, and graduated with honors. As the years passed, the pressures of his work as an accountant and the responsibility of a family stimulated him to smoke more and more. He read about the harmful effects of smoking and promised himself and his wife that he would quit smoking someday. He tried to quit once, but started again after a few days.

*In the case studies in this book, all names and some of the details have been changed to preserve confidentiality.

One weekend while playing basketball with his sons, Mr. Dawson noted a pain in his chest. The pain went away quickly when he stopped playing and returned when he resumed the game. He made an appointment to see his doctor the following Monday.

Dr. Johnson gave him a thorough examination and made a diagnosis of coronary heart disease. The chest X-ray that was taken showed a shadow—about an inch in diameter—in the upper part of the right lung. The doctor thought it might be a tumor even though there were none of the usual symptoms, such as cough, blood spitting, or shortness of breath. When Dr. Johnson compared the new X-ray film with one that had been made about two years earlier, he saw no abnormality in the older film.

Mr. Dawson could not believe he had cancer, but agreed to have a sputum test for cancer cells. The test was negative, but the doctor told him that cancer was still a possibility, pointing out that in some cases the sputum does not show the cancer cells. He advised a bronchoscopic examination and this, too, was negative.

Dr. Johnson explained that there was still a very great chance that the lesion was cancerous. He recommended consulting a surgeon, to consider removing the portion of the lung containing the lesion. Mr. Dawson was not willing to have an operation without proof of cancer, so Dr. Johnson arranged another test, a transthoracic needle aspiration biopsy. This time adenocarcinoma cells were found, which settled the diagnosis and convinced Mr. Dawson that he should consult the thoracic surgeon without further delay.

(This story continues at the end of Chapter 4.)

COMMENT

Millions of people began smoking cigarettes before the danger was fully realized. They became addicted to the nicotine in the smoke and were unable to "kick the habit." Many of these smokers worked with asbestos, which alone can cause lung cancer. But the effect of one does not simply add to the effect of the other; they multiply, so the combination is very serious.

The diagnosis of lung cancer is frequently made when a chest X-ray film is taken as part of a routine checkup or when a person consults a physician for another medical problem. About twenty percent of lung cancers are discovered this way. Perhaps all smokers, especially those in the cancer age group, should have frequent chest X-ray examinations to increase the chance of detecting lung cancers before they grow large enough to cause symptoms.

CHAPTER 4

The Role of Surgery in the Treatment of Lung Cancer

During the latter part of the nineteenth century and the first part of the twentieth century, many surgeons operated on patients with lung cancer to try to remove the tumor. They were almost always unsuccessful because of heavy bleeding, infection, or other complications.

One of the first successful modern operations for lung cancer was performed in 1933 by Dr. Edward D. Churchill, of Boston, Massachusetts. Dr. Churchill removed the middle and lower lobe of the patient's right lung. That same year, Dr. Evarts A. Graham, of St. Louis, Missouri, successfully removed the entire left lung from an obstetrician who had cancer. The patient was cured and was able to resume his practice of medicine. He outlived his surgeon who, ironically, died of lung cancer many years later.

After that, the surgical treatment of lung cancer continued to become safer and more successful. Now, thousands of patients have these operations every year, and many are cured. They live active, normal lives for many years thereafter.

When Surgery Is Used

Surgery is usually the best treatment when there is a good chance that the tumor can be completely removed. If tests and studies show that the tumor is confined to only one lung, then the affected part or even the entire lung can be removed. If the cancer has spread to the lymph nodes in or near that lung, the surgeon may still be able to remove all of the cancer.

Sometimes an operation can cure a cancer that has grown outward from the lung into a small part of the chest wall. In such a case, the cancerous tissue on the chest wall may be cut out along with the diseased lung. The operation does not leave a hole in the chest wall. The surgeon uses pieces of muscle and other tissue to cover the portion of the chest wall that has been removed.

When Surgery Is Not Used

Surgery is not used when the cancer has spread to the other lung because there would not be enough lung capacity left for breathing.

Surgery is usually not possible for a tumor that has grown from the lung into vital organs in the chest, such as the heart, esophagus (swallowing tube), trachea (windpipe), or large blood vessels. Also, surgery cannot cure lung cancer that has spread to the lymph nodes in the neck, to the opposite lung, or to other organs such as the liver, kidneys, or brain.

Surgery is seldom advised for small cell lung cancer because that type of cancer will have spread outside of the lung in almost all cases by the time the diagnosis is made.

The Decision to Operate

Despite the skills of today's surgical teams, and despite the great care they take, patients sometimes die from complications of the operation. Therefore, your doctors will not operate unless you stand a good chance of cure.

These are among the questions they will consider before recommending surgery:

Is your cancer of a cell type that can be cured by surgery?

Do all of the clues indicate that the cancer has not spread outside the lungs?

Are you in good enough physical condition to pull through a serious operation?

Will your good lung work well enough to let you be moderately active after some or all of your diseased lung has been removed?

Based on your chances for cure, is the operation worth the risk?

Types of Surgery

The three most common types of operations for treating lung cancer are thoracotomy, lobectomy, and pneumonectomy. Because thoracotomy may be combined with one of the other surgical procedures, the terms can be confusing.

A *thoracotomy* allows careful and complete examination of a lung and the area near it, to find out exactly where the tumor is located, how far it has spread, whether it is malignant, and whether it can be removed by surgery.

If the tumor can be removed, the surgeon will go ahead and take out enough lung tissue to get rid of all the cancer. This second part of the operation will be called a lobectomy, a bilobectomy, or a pneumonectomy, depending on how much lung tissue is removed.

A *lobectomy* is the removal of one lobe of a lung.

A *bilobectomy* is removal of two of the right lung's three lobes.

A *pneumonectomy* is the removal of an entire lung.

While one lung is being operated on, the other lung continues to function. Special equipment will be used to help your breathing and make sure that you get enough oxygen during the operation.

What Happens During the Operation

Thoracotomy involves opening up one side of the chest enough for the surgeons to see inside easily and work in the area where the lung is. The incision follows the curve of the ribs on one side, starting just below the shoulder blade in back, and continuing around to the front of the chest. All or part of one rib may be removed, or two ribs may be spread apart.

Although the surgeons gather as much information as they can about a tumor before the operation, some questions can be answered only by directly examining the diseased lung and the tissues around it. If they find nothing more than a single, small lump of tumor, for example, and if all other conditions are good, they will probably go ahead and remove all or part of the lung.

On the other hand, if they see that the cancer has gone too far to get it all out, they will almost always leave the lung as it is. In this case, they will rely on other forms of cancer treatment, such as radiotherapy and chemotherapy.

After the chest has been opened, the surgeons may snip out one or more pieces of diseased lung tissue or lymph nodes and have them rushed to the pathology laboratory for microscopic examination. Within minutes, a report will be sent back to the operating room that identifies the type of cancer and indicates if it has spread. The pathology report will give the surgical team information about the curabililty of the cancer, so they can then decide whether they should proceed with removal of part or all of the lung.

Occasionally, the surgeons do not have a choice as to what to do. For example, they may find during surgery that removing a lung is the only way to achieve a cure. But if previous tests of lung function have shown that the patient's remaining lung cannot do the job of breathing by itself, they cannot remove the lung. This is most common if the patient has emphysema of the lungs as well as the lung cancer.

Special Indications for Lung Removal

In a few life-threatening situations, surgeons may remove a lung even though the cancer has spread beyond the lung and cannot be totally removed. Some tumors, for example, cause serious bleeding. The patient may cough up a lot of blood and be in danger of bleeding to death. An emergency operation may even be necessary.

Sometimes tumors cause severe infection. A lung that is infected and full of pus may have to be removed to save the patient's life. In such cases, it is sometimes possible to destroy the remaining cancer with radiotherapy or chemotherapy or a combination of both.

What Happens After a Lung Is Removed

Surgery for lung cancer is major surgery, and recovery takes time. You will probably be in an intensive care unit in the hospital for a day or two and then in a regular hospital room for another week or so. During this time, you can gradually increase your activity so you will be able to take care of yourself when you go home. There may be some pain in your incision; if so, your doctor will give you medicine to control the pain. You will be encouraged to cough up the mucus in your bronchi to reduce the risk of pneumonia developing.

After you recover from the immediate effects of the operation, you will be able to gradually increase your activity, and in a few months you may be able to lead a very active life, walking and playing sports such as golf and swimming.

Almost all patients are able to resume normal sexual activities also.

Even if an entire lung is removed, the remaining lung should do the work of breathing for you. Patients with only one lung may lead an active life.

You may wonder about the space that will be left in your chest after lung removal. Most of it will eventually fill with body fluid and scar tissue, which is the body's way of filling an empty space. In addition, the lung on the other side may expand slightly. Your ribs may sink in a little, and the operated side of the chest may appear slightly smaller than the other side. But the difference will not be enough to be very apparent, especially with clothes on.

CASE REPORT: ROBERT DAWSON

(Continued from Chapter 3)

A few days after the sequence of events that led to the diagnosis of Robert Dawson's lung cancer (see story at end of Chapter 3), he had a consultation with Dr. Johnson, his personal physician, and the thoracic surgeon, Dr. Hill. The doctors again explained the nature of the cancer and the reasons Mr. Dawson should have an operation. They assured him that in spite of his history of smoking, the measurements of his lung function showed that he could be fully active after the operation. They admitted that his coronary heart disease increased the risk slightly, but since he had had the pain only after strenuous exercise, and his stress test was negative, the risk was minimal. The rest of his examination, including a complete physical and blood and urine tests, was negative.

The operation was performed a couple of days later, and there were no complications. Dr. Hill and his team of associates removed the upper lobe of the right lung along with the lymph nodes next to the main bronchus and samples of lymph nodes in the mediastinum. The surgical pathologist, Dr. Fields, studied the specimen carefully and reported that the tumor was an adenocarcinoma, 2.5 centimeters in diameter, and that it had been completely removed. All the lymph nodes were negative for metastatic cancer.

After Mr. Dawson recovered from the operation, Dr. Hill and Dr. Johnson explained to him that his cancer was classified T1 N0 M0 Stage 1. They said he had about seventy percent probability of being cured by the operation alone and they did not advise further treatment, such as radiotherapy or chemotherapy. They strongly recommended, however, that he have checkups every four months for the next five years, to detect any recurrence of the cancer or a second primary cancer. Mr. Dawson had already stopped smoking and the doctors emphasized that he should never resume the use of any form of tobacco.

He followed their advice and now, five years later, he is alive and well. He plans to continue the checkups twice a year for the rest of his life.

COMMENT

Mr. Dawson was lucky. Unfortunately, many patients with lung cancer do not discover they have the disease until the cancer grows and causes symptoms. At that stage of the disease, the treatment is frequently more complicated and is less successful.

CHAPTER 5

The Role of Radiotherapy in the Treatment of Lung Cancer

by Robert E. Lee, M.D.

Many patients with lung cancer will need radiotherapy at some time during their illness. Radiotherapy consists of directing a beam of high-energy rays at a tumor in order to destroy it. By injuring the cancer cells so that they cannot continue to multiply, the treatments stop tumor growth. The effect of the radiation builds up with each treatment.

Another kind of radiotherapy involves placing radioactive material into the body near or inside the tumor, to slow or halt tumor growth. The radioactive material can also be placed in the lumen of the trachea or bronchus.

You may hear radiotherapy referred to by a variety of terms: X-ray therapy, X-ray treatment, irradiation, radiation therapy, radiation treatment, and cobalt treatment. Although these words are used synonymously, the meanings of some of them are different. Irradiation, radiation therapy, and radiation treatment are general terms. X-ray therapy or X-ray treatment is given with an X-ray machine that produces X-rays when high-speed electrons strike a heavy metal target. Cobalt treatment utilizes gamma rays that are produced in the nucleus of decaying radioactive (cobalt-60) atoms in a cobalt machine.

Radiotherapy has advanced tremendously in recent years with the result that improved techniques and options are available for the treatment of lung cancer.

Background

Radiotherapy was first used to treat lung cancer in 1915. The machines available at that time generated only low-energy rays. Unfortunately, these low-energy X-rays deposit most of the energy just below the surface of the skin, and lung cancer is usually situated deep within the chest.

Some machines used radium, a radioactive element, to destroy the tumor. This type of equipment, with its more penetrating beams, was a forerunner of the cobalt machines we have today.

By the 1920s, scientists had developed more powerful X-ray machines. These generated medium-energy rays that delivered more penetrating beams. Finally, in the 1930s, scientists began developing equipment that emitted high-energy X-rays, which could deposit more energy deep in the body where most lung cancers are situated.

In 1933, surgery and radiation were combined for the first time to treat lung cancer. After successfully removing the cancer from a lung, surgeons implanted radioactive material into the lung. Now it is common to use combinations of radiotherapy, surgery, and chemotherapy.

Cobalt machines were first used to treat lung cancer in the 1950s. A decade later, they were joined by linear accelerators and other machines using millions of volts of energy. Recent advances in all these machines now permit radiation to be delivered to deeper tissues, with more precision than ever before.

Radiotherapy Equipment

The X-rays used for cancer treatment are similar to those that take pictures of the bones and organs of the body. The main difference is that in radiotherapy the dose is thousands of times larger, and the rays are thousands of times more powerful. Large doses of X-rays—especially when repeated —can damage or kill body tissues, and that is what makes X-rays effective against cancer.

Ideally, a large amount of radiation strikes the tumor and only a small zone of surrounding normal tissues. Doctors use the technique of aiming the X-ray beams at the tumor from several directions or angles, so that each beam takes a different pathway through normal tissue. This method enables the tumor to get a high enough dose of radiation to be destroyed, with minimum radiation effects on normal tissue.

Two types of machines are most often used to radiate lung cancer: the *linear accelerator* and the *cobalt machine*. Both of these give off high-energy rays that penetrate deeply into the body's tissues. Both machines also contain complex controls, safety devices, and mechanisms for directing the radiation beams at an exact location in a precise dose, so that very little normal tissue gets irradiated.

Their difference lies in their methods of producing the high-energy beams. The linear accelerator uses electricity, the same kind that comes from the electrical outlets in your home, except that the voltage is much higher. The X-rays are emitted from the electrons of the atom.

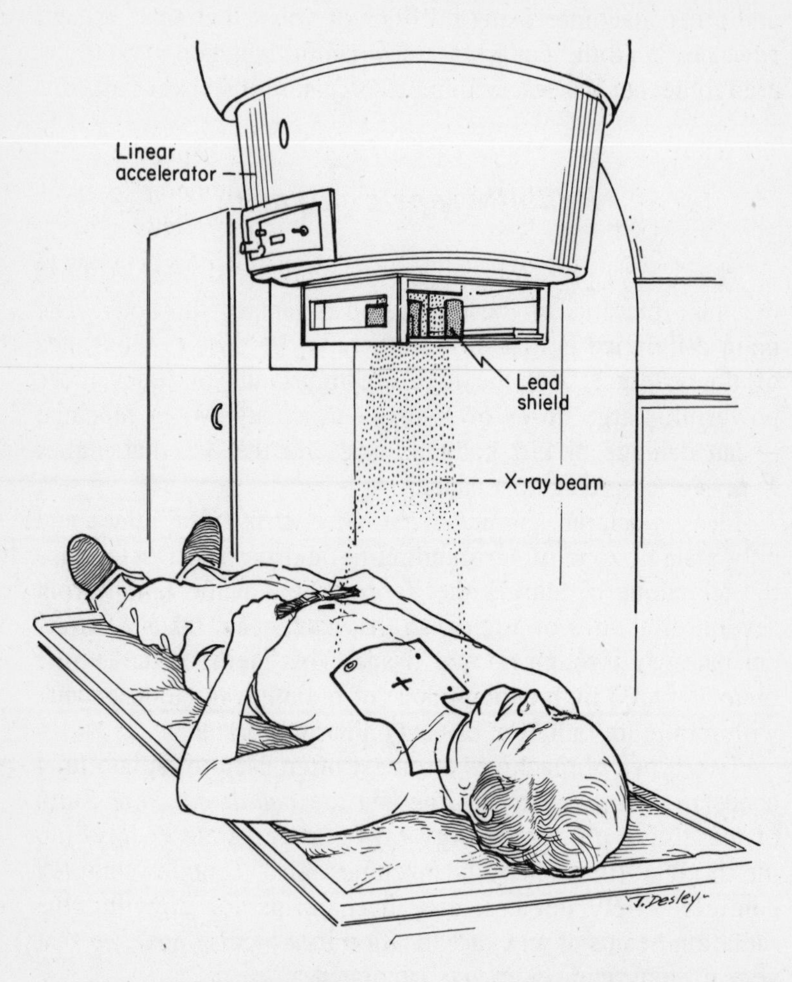

Patient receiving radiotherapy. He is lying on the treatment couch, and the beam from the linear accelerator above him is aimed at the left side of his chest and neck. The area to be treated is marked to include all of the cancer. A lead shield placed in the linear accelerator allows only the marked area to be treated, protecting the rest of the body from radiation. The X-ray beam is shown in this diagram but is is invisible to the patient.

The cobalt machine uses cobalt, a metal that can be made radioactive for the purpose of treating persons with cancer. The gamma rays are emitted from the nucleus of the atom. Although the cobalt's radioactivity cannot be turned on and off in the way that electrical power can, it does not affect the patient until the cobalt is moved into the proper position for radiotherapy.

Both the cobalt machine and the linear accelerator are extremely large. Although they may look frightening because of their size, most of their bulk consists of a safety feature—heavy shielding that prevents the escape of radiation when and where it is not wanted.

Treatment with Radiotherapy

In patients whose lung cancer has spread to vital organs such as the heart, esophagus, or large blood vessels, surgical removal will usually not be done. However, radiotherapy will often be beneficial. Some patients cannot tolerate an operation becaue they have other serious medical problems, such as a recent heart attack. In these cases, radiotherapy can be used and may be able to cure the cancer.

Treatment with Radiotherapy and Surgery

Surgeons do not recommend removing a patient's lung unless numerous tests indicate a good chance for a cure. Sometimes, however, they discover more cancer during the operation than the tests showed. There may be cancer cells in the lymph nodes, for example. They will probably remove these nodes, but they know from experience that if the lymph nodes are involved, some microscopic bits of cancer may remain in the chest. If so, radiotherapy may be planned for the part of the chest that is most likely to contain cancer cells. The patient probably will be given several weeks to rest so that the tissues heal before radiotherapy begins.

Occasionally surgery is considered even though the doctor knows that the tumor has spread beyond the lung. In that case, radiotherapy may be given before surgery, in hopes of shrinking the tumor so it can be removed more easily. Preoperative radiotherapy may alter the viability of tumor cells, decreasing the likelihood of local recurrence and distant dissemination of cancer. The surgery usually takes place three to four weeks after the course of radiotherapy is over and the patient has recovered from the radiation treatments.

Treatment with Radiotherapy and Chemotherapy

The doctors who specialize in treating cancer are still studying the possible benefits of combining radiotherapy and chemotherapy, and the most effective order of applying them. So far, they have found the combined therapy to be particulary useful in treating small cell carcinoma.

They may use radiotherapy first to destroy this radiosensitive tumor in the chest region, and follow it with chemotherapy. Most oncologists, however, start with chemotherapy and add radiotherapy later. They are then able to test whether chemotherapy alone is effective in shrinking the tumor. A smaller tumor is more likely to be controlled by radiotherapy (see chemotherapy chapter).

Prophylactic or *elective radiotherapy* is the term used to describe combined therapy in which radiotherapy is given to reduce the chance of metastatic new tumor growth, after chemotherapy has controlled most of the cancer cells in the body.

For example, suppose the doctor believes there is a good chance that small cell cancer cells will metastasize to the brain. Because the brain has a protective mechanism that does not allow certain chemicals to enter (a biological screen called the "blood-brain barrier"), chemotherapy may not be of any help. A drug may work in the lung, but it will not work in the brain if it does not cross the barrier. The doctor might suggest prophylactic brain radiotherapy in this case.

Studies of the effectiveness of chemotherapy combined with radiotherapy for lung cancers other than small cell carcinoma are being conducted, and there is some evidence of benefit.

Planning Your Treatment

If your doctor thinks you need radiation therapy, he or she will consult with a *radiation oncologist.* (Radiation oncologist, radiation therapist, radiotherapist, therapeutic radiologist are synonyms, but radiation oncologist is preferred.) The radiation oncologist will decide whether this treatment is advisable, and if so, which kind of radiation will be best for you, how much radiation you will need, and how often you should have treatments.

Sometimes the radiation oncologist will call on a *radiation physicist* if special measurements are needed (though not all departments of radiation oncology have a full-time radiation physicist).

A *dosimetrist* calculates the distribution of the doses of radiation you will be given and how the beams will be arranged. If you have radiotherapy, you will probably meet *radiation therapy nurses* and *technologists*. These people are trained to help in the care of patients and to assist the radiotherapist.

The goal of the radiotherapy team is to give you a dose of radiation that is high enough to kill the cancer cells but low enough to cause as few side effects as possible. The dose you are to be given is determined by the radiation oncologist. This total dose is then divided into a number of daily doses, or *fractions*. By the time the last treatment is reached, all of the fractions will add up to the total dose.

There is a good reason for dividing the radiation into small doses rather than giving it all at once. Even though the radiation is aimed at the cancer cells, it also causes some unavoidable damage to the normal cells in the immediate area. Because normal cells recover more quickly than cancer cells, treating with a small dose of radiation allows the normal cells to recover between treatments. If the total dose were given all at once, many normal cells would be damaged beyond repair.

To calculate the radiation distribution in the chest area, the dosimetrist or technologist begins by making a kind of map or outline, called a *contour*, of the portion of your chest that is to be treated, and then calculates the dose distribution of the intersecting beams in the tumor region, taking into account your specific anatomy. Some departments of radiation oncology have computers that are used in making these calculations.

Treatment schedules vary from one doctor to the another. The most commonly used schedule consists of daily treatments for five to seven weeks. Another might call for daily treatments for one to three weeks, a "rest" period of two to four weeks, followed by a second course of daily treatments over the next one to three weeks. Sometimes three courses of radiotherapy are used with rest periods between the courses. The cure rate for each of these schedules is equally good.

Locating the Tumor

A combination of fluoroscopy and simulation films are used to find the exact location of a tumor. Fluoroscopy is an examination in which X-rays pass through the body and project the X-ray image on a screen. Simulation films are X-rays taken with a special diagnostic X-ray machine (simulator) using the exact field size, treatment distance, and angle that will be used for therapy.

When the area to be treated is found on these X-rays, the radiotherapist or technologist draws an outline on your skin with a special marking pen. Then this location is double-checked by making a "port film," which is an X-ray made with the treatment machine. With the tumor outlined, the beam can be aimed at exactly the same spot each time. You will be asked not to wash the outline off until your radiotherapy treatments are finished. Often a tiny tattoo is made to mark the spot permanently.

What Happens During Radiation Treatments

When you are receiving radiation, you will be brought into a treatment room that contains a couch and an enormous X-ray or cobalt machine. To protect the normal tissue around the tumor from the radiation beam, the radiotherapist or technician places a shielding device over you to shape the treatment beam. Your shield will be made especially for you, and will be either a single piece of lead molded to the size and shape of your tumor region, or lead shields arranged on a wire mesh or plastic tray to fit the size and shape of this region. Either way, the shield will be held securely in place between you and the X-ray machine.

You will be asked to lie on the couch. Then the couch and the machine will be moved until the right position is reached. Care will be given to beam the radiation at the exact part of the lung where the cancer is, so that as little normal tissue as possible is affected. The machine must be correctly positioned in relation to your chest, and about twelve inches away. The equipment does not touch you.

As soon as the radiation specialists are sure that the beam is aimed accurately and the controls are properly adjusted, they leave and go to a control room. They are not allowed to stay in the room with you because, even though their exposure to radiation would be tiny during any one treatment session, over the years it would add up to a dangerous amount.

Patients who do not understand the procedure are sometimes alarmed at being left alone. However, you are alone for only a few minutes, and you are never out of touch with the staff. An intercom system lets you talk with the people in the control room, and a closed circuit television system between the treatment room and control room lets the staff watch you at all times.

When the treatment starts, you will hear a soft whirring or buzzing sound. Each treatment lasts only a few minutes. There is no physical discomfort. In fact, you will feel no sensation that anything is happening. The radiotherapy staff returns immediately afterward.

Your treatments will be given from different directions or from different angles. Therefore, you may receive treatments through the front and back of your chest or from two different directions each day. If only one treatment a day were used, the normal tissues near the surface of the chest overlying the lung tumor would receive a greater dose than the tumor. Therefore, for cancer deep in the chest, two or more areas are treated daily to spare normal tissues.

How Radiotherapy Affects the Lung

In the days and weeks after radiation treatment, the lung gradually changes. Radiation injury of the cancer and surrounding lung causes inflammatory changes in the irradiated lung called *radiation pneumonitis.* Though these changes can be seen on X-rays taken two to six months after therapy, they usually do not cause any discomfort or symptoms.

About a year after radiotherapy, scar tissue forms in the lung. If the radiation treatment has been given to an entire lung, that lung is no longer able to function normally, so the lung on the other side takes over the job of meeting the body's need for oxygen. Most people are able to adjust well to the lower lung capacity, although they must usually cut down on their physical activities.

Some patients with lung cancer also have emphysema, a condition of the lung characterized by air-filled expansions with impairment of function. Radiotherapy does not help emphysema. In fact, the scar tissue due to radiation therapy can make the problem worse.

Side Effects

Tiredness

A feeling of general tiredness is the most common side effect of radiotherapy for lung cancer, and it usually occurs within a few hours of the treatment. During the course of daily treatments, you may feel tired most of the time. You should rest and take naps if you can. And you should not expect to get much done during this period. This tiredness generally starts to wear off about a week after treatments end.

Skin Reactions

In the early days of radiotherapy for lung cancer, most patients suffered severe inflammation and skin reactions in the treated area. Now, with engineering advances and more sophisticated equipment, the side effects of radiation on the skin are minimal.

Usually the skin in the treated area becomes slightly pink a few days after treatment. Then it tans slightly, turns a bit rough, and perhaps peels a little. The skin may not be quite as movable or flexible as it was before.

To take care of irradiated skin, you should keep it protected from the sun. Avoid using harsh ointments or medicines (like mustard plaster), and do not apply a heating pad. However, a mild, soothing skin lotion such as baby oil is often helpful in making the skin more smooth and comfortable.

Sore or Dry Throat

Within a few days to two weeks after radiation treatments, you may notice dryness and soreness of the throat. You may also have some trouble swallowing. Food may seem to "stick."

This problem is frightening to some patients, who fear that the cancer is growing in their throats. But it is not. The symptoms are just some of the temporary side effects of radiotherapy, caused by radiation irritating the tissues in the throat and swallowing tube. The discomfort seldom lasts more than a week. Drink liquids and eat soft foods until the problem clears up. Suggested foods can be found in the chapter on nutrition.

Fever and Coughing

The most common symptoms of radiation pneumonitis are mild fever and coughing. If you should have these symptoms, your doctor can prescribe medicine to make you more comfortable and control any infection that may develop.

Hair Loss

Men who have much hair on their chests will find that the hair in the treated area falls out within a few weeks after treatment. It may grow back after about three months, although it will be a little thinner.

Stiff Muscles

In a few patients, the chest and shoulder muscles on the treated side harden slightly about a year after treatment. These muscles may ache a little and be slightly stiff. You can minimize this problem by exercising daily; it would be a good idea to begin while you are still getting treatments. Start with your arms stretched out to the side and then bring them gradually upward, until your hands meet above your head. Lock your fingers briefly while your arms are stretched upward. Then slowly lower your arms to your sides again. Do this several times a day.

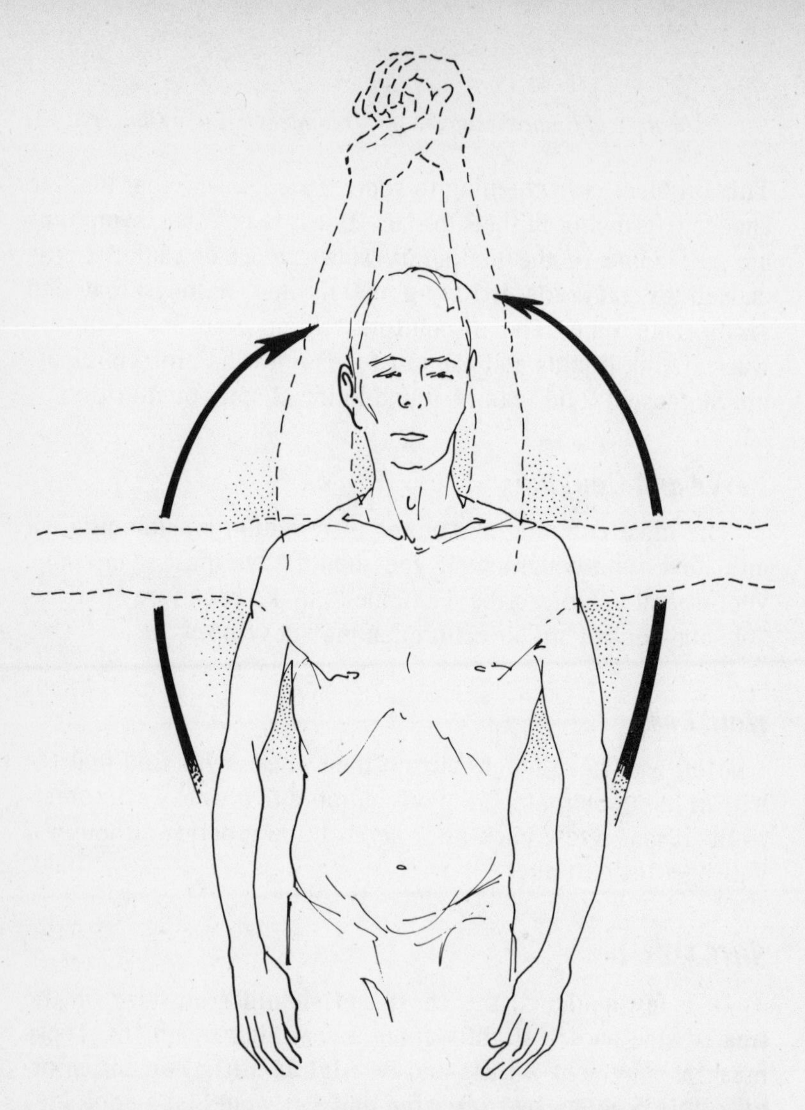

Exercise that prevents stiffness of the muscles and limitation of motion in the shoulder joint. Because radiotherapy to the chest can damage the muscles of the chest and shoulder, patients should exercise these muscles several times a day. The arms should be raised slowly from the sides until they are stretching out from the body. Then they should be raised until they are straight above the head so that the fingers can be locked together. Finally, the arms should be lowered slowly to the sides.

Nausea

Some patients having radiotherapy to the chest will have nausea. When this happens, it may well be related to chemotherapy they are getting at the same time. Medication can be given to relieve the nausea.

Palliative Radiotherapy

Radiotherapy that is done to shrink tumors in order to relieve symptoms is called *palliative radiotherapy*. In the lung, these symptoms may be coughing, spitting up of blood, and chest pain. Palliative radiotherapy is also done to relieve symptoms when cancer has spread to other parts of the body.

In the lymph nodes, a tumor is usually painless as long as the nodes are small. But as the cancer cells multiply, the nodes can get bigger and may press on nerves, causing pain and stopping the nerves from functioning properly. Radiotherapy can shrink the nodes to get rid of the pain, or at least lessen it.

A metastatic tumor in the brain can cause headache, nausea, vomiting, double vision, weakness of an arm or leg, or other problems. A course of radiotherapy usually relieves these symptoms. Shrinking the tumor in the brain takes enough pressure off the brain tissue so that it can function more or less normally again.

Metastatic cancer in bones usually causes pain. After radiotherapy, the metastases shrink and the pain usually goes away. Radiotherapy can also help to avoid a fracture in a bone weakened by cancer.

Sometimes radiotherapy can save your life. When a tumor blocks an essential blood vessel, closes off the swallowing tube, or presses on the windpipe, radiation treatments can shrink the tumor enough to stop dangerous symptoms. Radiotherapy can also stop heavy bleeding caused by a lung tumor.

Radiotherapy is seldom used for metastatic lung cancer in organs such as the liver or kidneys. Tumors in these organs are hard to treat without damaging the normal tissues, since the normal tissue is usually more sensitive to radiation than the cancer.

Radiotherapy cannot be given to a lung if the opposite lung has been removed by surgery or damaged by previous radiotherapy. The patient would not have enough lung tissue left for breathing.

Self-Care During Radiotherapy

Taking good care of yourself during radiotherapy means eating well and getting plenty of rest. This is particularly important if you are getting chemotherapy at the same time. Both kinds of therapy destroy large numbers of cells in the body—not only cancer cells, but normal cells. You need a diet with enough calories to keep up your weight, enough protein to rebuild damaged cells, and a proper supply of vitamins.

Rest, too, helps your body muster its strength and repair itself. By resting, you put your energy reserves into recovery. What energy you do have should be devoted to work that you enjoy or to recreation, if possible.

Radiotherapy can offer you greater comfort and a better quality of life. Sometimes it can cure the disease altogether. When it cannot solve a particular problem, the physician has other means to help you. These are discussed in other chapters of the book.

CASE REPORT: THOMAS WILLIAMSON

Thomas Wlliamson, an insurance salesman, had a pneumonectomy for a large squamous cell carcinoma of his left lung. The diagnosis had been made by Dr. Thornton, his personal physician, when he had consulted him for a cigarette cough that had gradually worsened.

After the operation, Dr. Thornton and the surgeon, Dr. Hamilton, told Mr. Williamson that the cancer had spread from the lung to the lymph nodes adjacent to the left main bronchus. However, the lymph nodes from the mediastinum had no cancer cells in them. They classified his cancer as T2 N1 M0 Stage 2, and explained that there was no definite evidence that he had any residual cancer. Nevertheless, they offered him a program of experimental postoperative radiotherapy and chemotherapy, and described the side effects of the chemotherapy and the possible benefit that he would get from the treatment.

When he asked about alternatives, he was told that he could have frequent checkups and treatment as needed if the cancer ever caused more trouble. After thinking about the benefits and the risks, Mr. Williamson decided not to have the experimental treatment, but he arranged to have the checkup examinations.

He got along very well until about two years later, when, after a game of golf, he became aware of pain in his lower back. Aspirin relieved the pain at first, but gradually it worsened until it began to waken him during the night.

He returned to Dr. Thornton, who arranged for X-ray films of his back. These showed that he had metastatic cancer in one of the bones in his back. Dr. Rodriguez, a specialist in radiotherapy, was called in consultation and recommended a course of radio-

therapy. The treatment relieved the backache completely. Although a thorough examination revealed no other metastases, Mr. Williamson was again offered the experimental chemotherapy. He again elected to have only routine checkups.

Mr. Williamson continues to work, and he has an active life that includes playng golf twice a week.

COMMENT

Mr. Williamson understands that he may have metastases to other bones and other organs such as the liver. He has carefully considered the possible benefit of chemotherapy and the side effects of the drugs and has decided to wait and have more treatment when and if there is definite evidence of active metastatic cancer. When chemotherapy, or other systemic treatment, becomes less toxic and more certain to control all microscopic metastases, all patients like Mr. Williamson will be urged to take it without waiting for proof that the cancer has spread.

CHAPTER 6

The Role of Chemotherapy in the Treatment of Lung Cancer

Chemotherapy means the "treatment of disease by drugs." Technically, it includes even the treatment of a headache with aspirin. In actual usage, however, chemotherapy usually refers to the treatment of malignant tumors with cancer-killing drugs. There are presently about a dozen chemotherapy drugs used to treat lung cancer.

Background

Before World War II, there was little interest in using chemotherapy for treating cancer, and very few scientists were working on the problem. During the war, however, several factors stimulated interest in chemotherapy as a treatment for cancer.

One was an incident in which a ship carrying mustard gas was blown up, exposing the men to the poison and killing many of them. When chemical warfare experts discovered that the white blood cells and lymph nodes of the dead men had been destroyed by the mustard gas, they suspected that mustard gas or similar chemicals might be of value in treating certain types of cancer.

About the same time, a group of scientists discovered that nitrogen mustard was effective against a certain cancerous growth in mice. They then began to study its use in patients with cancer.

Another factor that sparked interest in chemotherapy was the phenomenal success of penicillin, and the discovery of other antibiotics and chemicals in the treatment of infections.

The search for anti-cancer drugs grew rapidly after World War II. Although a number of effective drugs were discovered, scientists learned there was no single drug that could combat every form of cancer. They also discovered that combinations of two or more drugs were frequently better than any single drug.

These lessons have been applied to the search for effective chemotherapy for lung cancer. Although much has been learned, a great deal more research must still be done before we have drugs that are as effective against lung cancer as the drugs used to treat other lung diseases, such as pneumonia and tuberculosis. Most of the chemotherapy for lung cancer must still be done in the form of carefully controlled experimental studies, so that their value can be measured. Whenever programs of treatment prove to be effective, they continue to be used; those that don't work are terminated.

How Chemotherapy Works

Because cancer cells usually grow more rapidly than normal cells, they are more prone to damage and destruction by drugs. Chemotherapy drugs, designed to kill cancer cells, may cure the cancer or at least control the growth of the tumor.

Different drugs attack cancer cells in different ways. Some destroy the reproductive capacity of the cells. Some disrupt the growth cycle. Some are chemically similar to the food needed by the cells but do not actually provide nourishment, so the cells starve. Doctors have found that they can take advantage of the many ways the drugs attack cancer cells by using more than one drug and varying the intervals between treatments.

You may wonder why you aren't getting the same treatment as another patient you have met. Drug treatment programs are tailored to the needs of each individual. Doctors cannot always predict what the effect of a drug will be on any given patient. The chemotherapy that helps one patient fails to stop tumor growth in another.

Your chemotherapy treatment plan takes into account the kind of lung cancer you have, how widespread it is, your state of general health, and other medical considerations. You are not limited to the first drug treatment recommended for you. If one drug fails, another may be tried. Sometimes a drug stops working because the cancer cells have become resistant to it. Another drug may then provide good results. Or another form of treatment may be given.

Treatment with Chemotherapy

The most common use of chemotherapy in lung cancer is for attacking cancer cells that have spread to other sites in the body. Because these drugs go into the bloodstream, they may control new tumor growth anywhere that tumor cells might be growing.

In the very fortunate patient, chemotherapy can cause the lung cancer to disappear altogether. Even if the chemotherapy doesn't destroy all the cancer cells, it may control your cancer until a new drug or treatment can be found. Since new treatments are constantly being developed, your chances for more effective treatment continue to improve.

Treatment with Chemotherapy and Surgery

When chemotherapy is used in combination with surgery, it is called "adjuvant therapy," meaning that it has been "added to" the surgery. Sometimes drugs are used after surgery as a preventive measure. For example, a patient may have had a lung removed with the expectation that the operation would cure the cancer. The surgeons cannot see any cancer cells remaining nor do they have any evidence based on laboratory tests. But if the oncologist still suspects that microscopic clusters of cancer cells remain in the chest, chemotherapy will be recommended to prevent a recurrence.

In other cases, chemotherapy is given before surgery, to shrink the tumor. The smaller tumor is then easier to remove, making the chance of cure better.

Effective drugs have not yet been identified for every type of lung cancer, so adjuvant chemotherapy is not always useful. However, as research continues, more and more effective chemotherapy drugs are being discovered.

Treatment with Chemotherapy and Radiotherapy

Chemotherapy used in combination with radiotherapy is sometimes more effective than either treatment alone. The chemotherapy is given over a period of several months, followed by a course of radiation treatments.

Scientists are working on a new kind of drug treatment called *radiosensitization.* Drugs are administered that, by themselves, would not kill cancer cells, but are thought to make the cancer cells more sensitive to radiotherapy.

How Chemotherapy Is Given

The drugs for treating lung cancer can be given in several ways: as pills or capsules, as shots, or intravenously (directly into the bloodstream). The frequency of treatment varies from daily to weekly to monthly, depending on the drugs being used and how quickly you recover from the side effects. Most doctors prefer giving chemotherapy on an outpatient basis in their office or in a clinic. Being treated as an outpatient is more economical than being admitted to the hospital, and it enables you to be at home with your family.

Although people usually prefer taking their medication by mouth, most chemotherapy drugs cannot be given that way. Many of the drugs are destroyed by stomach acid, and others simply are not well absorbed by the stomach and therefore cannot reach the bloodstream.

In most cases, the drugs will be given intravenously. The "infusion" method is commonly used. With this method, the drug is mixed with fluid, hung in an IV (intravenous) bag, and allowed to drip slowly into an arm vein. In other cases the drug may be given in only a few minutes using a syringe and a needle.

If your chemotherapy is given intravenously and must be injected frequently or continuously for several days, your doctor may insert a catheter in one of your veins and leave it in place for the entire treatment time. The vein selected may be in your arm or near your collarbone. You will be instructed by the doctor or nurse in the care of the catheter to reduce the risk of infection and to prevent blood from clotting in the catheter.

If chemotherapy is to be given over a period of twenty-four hours or longer, a pump may be used to get the medicine through the catheter and into your bloodstream at the proper rate. You will be given instructions in the care of the pump.

Experimental Treatment Programs

All major hospitals have experimental chemotherapy programs—called "drug protocols"—available for patients with lung cancer. Every drug has been extensively tested before it is given to patients and the protocol will have been approved by a medical review committee concerned with patients' safety and rights.

Before experimental drugs are ever used on patients, each is first tested on animals with tumors similar to those found in humans. Since animals and humans have many similar organs and body functions, drugs that have proved effective against animal tumors often work well against human tumors. In testing, some animals receive a drug treatment and some do not. For a drug to be tried in humans, scientists must first prove that the treated animals live significantly longer than the untreated ones.

The scientists then design treatment programs for people with specific kinds of cancer, taking into account the many differences between animals and humans, such as weight and size. Only a small number of patients can participate in the first trials of a drug, called Phase 1 studies. If the pilot studies show that the drug is safe and effective, the treatment program is offered to larger numbers of patients in Phase 2 and Phase 3 studies.

Many drug protocols for lung cancer use drug combinations instead of individual drugs, because doctors need to learn which combinations will be the most effective.

Some patients mistakenly get the idea that new experimental drugs are not as safe and effective as nonexperimental ones. Actually, they may be safer and more effective than the older drugs. The research is designed to determine if the new drug is better.

Experimental drug protocols are coordinated on a nationwide basis by the National Cancer Institute. All of the findings are pooled, providing a large enough research base to give doctors a clearer view of how well a drug works.

When a new drug or drug combination is shown to work as well as or better than other chemotherapy drugs, the evidence is presented at medical meetings and published in medical journals. In that way, all physicians who treat cancer patients have access to the most up-to-date information.

Participating in Research

You should discuss your options for treatment with your doctor. It's important for you to understand all the different possibilities. If you want to consider taking part in a drug protocol program, ask your doctor if you are eligible and what drugs will be given. Your doctor will determine whether you meet the requirements of any of the programs being used by considering your general health as well as the type and extent of your cancer.

If you decide to participate in a protocol, you will be given information about the goals of the treatment protocol, drugs to be used, how the drugs act, and what side effects you can expect. Then you will be asked to sign a consent form that states that you have had all of these factors explained to you. You should ask all the questions you have before signing the consent form.

There are several advantages to being in a research protocol. The main one is the possibility that the drugs will shrink the tumor better than other available treatments. Also, many patients feel good about being part of a study that will help scientists learn more about fighting cancer.

Any time you wish to withdraw from a protocol, for any reason, you may. Some patients are concerned that withdrawing from a protocol will upset their doctor. They worry that the doctor will no longer try to help them. This almost never happens. Your doctors recognize the importance of your willingness to receive treatment and will respect your wishes.

Side Effects of Chemotherapy

It may take weeks or months before the benefits of chemotherapy become apparent. In the meantime, you may feel worse than you did before, especially after each treatment. It may be helpful to know that as you are having some uncomfortable side effects from the treatment, your tumor may be shrinking.

The goal of chemotherapy is to make you feel better in the long run, and to provide a longer, more meaningful life. In general, you should be as active as possible during and after chemotherapy. Moderate exercise, such as walking or swimming, is beneficial to your overall well-being.

Some side effects may be unavoidable, because what is effective about chemotherapy—that it attacks the fast-growing cancer cells—is also what causes side effects. Chemotherapy damages certain normal body cells that also grow rapidly. Examples of fast-growing cells that may be affected are the bone marrow, the lining of the digestive tract, and the hair follicles. Fortunately, normal cells can repair themselves, so most of the effects are only temporary.

Whether you experience one or more of the many possible side effects will depend on (1) the particular drugs you are getting, (2) your individual reaction to them, and (3) the dosage. Some patients have few or no side effects. Most have a limited number of side effects. Your doctor can tell you which side effects you are likely to experience. However, his prediction can only be general, because different people react so differently to any given drug.

The following are the most common side effects. Knowing what they are ahead of time may help you understand them as they develop.

Tiredness

People receiving chemotherapy often feel tired throughout treatment. The tiredness usually subsides a few days after the last treatment. You may have to nap during the day and go to bed earlier than usual.

No one knows the reason for the tiredness. It may be caused by the general stress that chemotherapy puts on your body. In part it may be from the reduction in the number of red blood cells brought about by chemotherapy. Red blood cells carry oxygen to all parts of your body, and when you don't get enough oxygen, you feel tired.

Nausea and Vomiting

Many drugs cause nausea, often with vomiting. This side effect may occur anytime from several minutes to several hours after the drugs are given, and it usually disappears within twenty-four to forty-eight hours. If you have chemotherapy daily over a period of several days, you may feel nauseous from the time of your first treatment until a day after the last treatment.

Not all chemotherapy drugs cause these symptoms. If your treatment is one that is likely to cause nausea and vomiting, your doctor will know and will prescribe medicine that may prevent or reduce the problem. Anti-nausea medicines may be given by injection or in the form of pills, liquids, or rectal suppositories.

Hair Loss

Some patients lose their hair, either partially or totally. Hair loss may occur on both the head and body, and includes eyelashes, eyebrows, mustaches, and beards. Sometimes, instead of falling out, the hair may change color and texture.

Hair loss occurs because the hair follicles grow rapidly and therefore are vulnerable to anti-cancer drugs. The hair usually falls out two to three weeks after treatment, over a period of several days, or it may thin gradually. It usually grows back when the drugs are stopped, although it may be slightly different in texture and color than it was before. Men who had mustaches and beards will find that facial hair seems to grow back faster than the hair on the head.

Some patients are not bothered by hair loss. Others find it hard to accept. If hair loss is a possible side effect of your treatment, you may want to purchase a wig in advance. Then you will be able to match your hair color. Your hair may take anywhere from three or four months to a year to grow back.

Wigs are a tax-deductible medical expense when hair loss is the result of chemotherapy.

Mouth Sores

The tissues inside your mouth are made of cells that grow rapidly, and therefore they can be affected by anti-cancer drugs. When mouth problems occur, they usually start a few days after the first treatment and range from a minor irritation to severe mouth sores.

With a minor irritation, your mouth may be sensitive to spicy foods, certain acid-containing foods such as fruit, or foods that are very hot or cold. Any of these may cause discomfort.

With a severe reaction, you may have tender open places in your mouth. Though these can be quite painful, they do heal a few days after chemotherapy has stopped. Your doctor may prescribe medication to ease the discomfort and also prevent infection. It is important to keep up good mouth care.

It may be tempting to stop brushing and flossing your teeth, but doing that can result in infection, which would aggravate the soreness of your mouth and throat.

Diarrhea

Some patients get diarrhea on the days of their treatment or shortly thereafter. It usually disappears within a few days after treatment has been stopped. If you have diarrhea, you should tell your doctor, who may prescribe a medicine to control it.

Lowered Blood Count

Most of the body's blood cells are made in the bone marrow. Because they grow rapidly, they are susceptible to chemotherapy. The side effects that drug treatments can have on the bone marrow usually don't become evident until a couple of weeks after the treatment. The blood cells are of three types: red blood cells, white blood cells, and platelets. The side effects from chemotherapy for each are different and usually don't become evident until a couple of weeks or longer after the treatment begins.

Red blood cells (RBCs). After many courses of chemotherapy, your RBC level may slowly fall, causing you to become anemic. Anemia means that there are not enough RBCs to carry oxygen to all the tissues of the body. Its main symptom is continual tiredness, for which your doctor may recommend extra rest and sleep, and possibly a blood transfusion. When the drug treatments are over, the RBCs return to normal levels.

White blood cells (WBCs). Because white blood cells help fight infection, lowered levels of WBCs make you more susceptible to various infections. Although the level can fall below normal without great danger, it is important for your doctor to keep track of your WBCs by means of a blood test about once a week. To help fight infections, your doctor may suggest antibiotics, a flu shot, or a pneumonia vaccine. During chemotherapy, you should avoid people who have contagious illnesses. If you should show signs of infection, such as a fever of 101 degrees or more, you should call your doctor right away.

Platelets. These are very small cells that help prevent bleeding. If your platelet count drops very low because of chemotherapy, you may notice a tendency to bleed easily and find that a cut takes a long time to stop bleeding. You may get nosebleeds or bleeding gums, or begin to bruise easily. Or you may notice clusters of tiny red spots just under the skin, called *petechiae.* They are tiny blood vessels that have broken. Your doctor will want to know about any of these.

Regular blood tests will be done so your doctor can monitor your platelets. If the platelet count gets low, you will need to avoid activities that might result in cuts or bruises. You should also avoid taking any medicine containing aspirin unless it has been prescribed.

Skin Irritation

A few chemotherapy drugs may cause itching, mild scaling of the skin, or skin rashes. The irritation generally disappears when the drug is stopped. If the skin problem is very troublesome, your doctor may prescribe a skin medication.

Numbness and Tingling of Hands and Feet

Some chemotherapy drugs may affect the nerve endings, causing mild numbness and tingling in the hands and feet.

This seldom causes any problems, but if you have these symptoms, you should keep your doctor informed. If it gets severe enough that the function of your hands and feet seems impaired in some way, your doctor will probably stop giving the drug responsible for this reaction.

Bladder Irritation

If the drugs you are taking leave the body by way of the urine, they become concentrated in the urine and irritate the bladder. The result is a continual feeling of a need to urinate. You may be advised to drink lots of fluids, especially during the treatment period, to increase the quantity of urine and thereby decrease drug concentration. This reduces the irritation of the bladder.

Other Side Effects

As more new drugs are developed, other side effects will undoubtedly accompany them. If you have any new, puzzling problems after your chemotherapy begins, you should discuss them with your doctor. It's a good idea to jot down your questions so you won't forget them.

In fact, you should tell your doctor about any side effect or symptom that is troubling you. Most doctors are anxious to help you understand your illness and its treatment as fully as possible.

Drugs Used for Treatment of Lung Cancer

Following is a description of some drugs used to treat patients with lung cancer, how they are given, and their side effects.

Cisplatinum

This drug is also called Platinol and Cisplatin. It is given by intravenous infusion.

Early side effects may be nausea and vomiting during treatment and for four to twelve hours after the infusion is completed.

Late side effects may include a drop in blood cell counts seven to fourteen days after treatment, temporary hair loss or thinning beginning several weeks after treatment, and a change in your hearing of high-pitched sounds. It may damage the kidneys, causing an increase in urea and creatinine in the blood.

Cyclophosphamide

This drug is also called Cytoxan. It may be given intravenously or, rarely, by mouth.

Early side effects may be mild nausea, vomiting, and appetite loss. There may also be a sensation of sinus congestion when the drug is given intravenously.

Late side effects include a drop in blood cell counts seven to ten days after treatment, temporary hair loss two to three weeks after treatment, and bladder irritation, sometimes with blood in the urine.

Doxorubicin

This drug is also called Adriamycin. It is given intravenously.

Early side effects may include nausea and vomiting, a change in color of the urine to pink, orange, or red, and mild fever (less than 101 degrees) on the day of treatment.

Late side effects may include a drop in blood cell counts seven to ten days after treatment, mouth sores one to four days after treatment, temporary hair loss two to three weeks after treatment, and nail changes such as white streaks or loosening of the nails. Heart problems are possible after a long period of treatment, so periodic heart tests are done.

Etoposide

This drug is also called VP-16. It is given intravenously.

Early side effects may include mild nausea, vomiting, and appetite loss, and allergic reactions such as fever and rash.

Late side effects may include a drop in blood cell counts seven to fourteen days after treatment.

Fluorouracil

This drug is also called 5-fluorouracil, 5-FU, Adriacil, and Efudex. It is given intravenously.

Early side effects may include mild nausea, vomiting, and appetite loss.

Late side effects may include a drop in blood cell counts seven to twenty-one days after treatment, mouth sores within several days of treatment, temporary hair loss or thinning beginning several weeks after treatment, and diarrhea (which can be controlled by medication).

Methotrexate

This drug is given intravenously or, less often, by mouth.

Early side effects may include mild nausea and vomiting.

Late side effects may include decreased blood cell counts four to ten days after treatment, mouth sores two to seven days after treatment, skin rash on trunk and neck one to three days after treatment, and hair loss or thinning two to three weeks after treatment.

Mitomycin

This drug is also called Mutamycin or Mitomycin-C. It is given intravenously.

Early side effects may include nausea, vomiting, and appetite loss, and a mild fever (less than 101 degrees) on the day of treatment.

Late side effects may include a drop in blood cell counts three to six weeks after treatment.

Procarbazine

This drug is also called Matulane. It is given by mouth or by intravenous infusion.

Early side effects may include nausea and vomiting, and skin rashes and itching.

Late side effects may include decreases in blood cell counts, restlessness, drowsiness, and numbness and tingling sensations.

Vincristine

This drug is also called Oncovin. It is given intravenously.

Early side effects may include mild nausea, vomiting and appetite loss.

Late side effects may include temporary hair loss two to three weeks after treatment, numbness and tingling in the fingers and toes, and mild constipation with abdominal cramping within fourteen days.

Vinblastine

This drug is also called Velban. It is given intravenously.

Early side effects may include mild nausea, vomiting and appetite loss.

Late side effects may include a drop in blood cell counts, mouth sores, temporary hair loss two to three weeks after treatment, numbness and tingling in the fingers and toes, and mild constipation with abdominal cramping within fourteen days.

Other drugs are being added to the list for experimental use and may be recommended by your doctor. If your doctor suggests another drug, ask how it will be given, what side effects may develop, and how much is known about its effectiveness against your type of cancer.

CASE REPORT: ANTHONY BRYANT

Anthony Bryant is a truck driver who smoked two to three packs of cigarettes a day for many years. Although he tried to quit several times, driving long distances was frequently boring, and it was during long drives that he always started smoking again.

One morning while shaving, Mr. Bryant noticed a little lump above his right collarbone. It did not hurt so he ignored it. A week later, he thought it was a little larger, so he went to a medical clinic in his hometown. He was assigned to Dr. Hansen, who asked him a lot of questions, examined him from head to toe, and arranged for X-rays, blood tests, and sputum tests.

When Mr. Bryant returned to the clinic a few days later, Dr. Hansen explained that the chest X-ray film showed a typical picture of cancer in the right lung, with metastases to the lymph nodes in the mediastinum. Two specimens of sputum showed cancer cells of the small cell variety. Dr. Hansen explained that the lump above the right collarbone was also typical of a metastasis to the lymph nodes in that area. He added that there was no evidence that the cancer had spread to any other place.

Mr. Bryant was referred to the department of oncology in a large medical center, where he was examined by Dr. Martin, a medical oncologist, and Dr. Blackman, a therapeutic radiologist. The two doctors made the same diagnosis as Dr. Hansen had: small cell lung cancer with metastases to the mediastinal lymph nodes and the right supraclavicular lymph node. Their recommendation was that Mr. Bryant enter a research program that included intensive chemotherapy using four anti-cancer drugs, to be combined later with radiotherapy to the chest and brain. The treatment to the brain was advised even though there was no evidence of metastasis to the brain, because such metastatic tumors are common. They may be too small to be seen on CT scans of the brain, and the drugs used in chemotherapy do not get into the brain tissue very well.

After thinking about his problem and getting answers to all his questions about the side effects of the treatment, the possibility of his being cured by the treatment, and its cost, Mr. Bryant decided to enter the research program and signed all the consent papers.

The treatments took up a great deal of Mr. Bryant's time, but he was able to continue working part of the time between treatments. Mr. Bryant had what is called a complete response to therapy. The lesion in his lung cleared up, and both the mediastinal lymph nodes and the one above his right collarbone returned to normal.

One year after the diagnosis, he feels fine and is working full time. He has regular checkups because he knows there is a possibility of having more trouble in the future. Needless to say, he has stopped smoking and now urges all of his friends to quit before they have trouble.

COMMENT

Mr. Bryant is one of the lucky patients with small cell lung cancer who seems to have been cured by the combination of chemotherapy and radiotherapy. Unfortunately, all patients with this disease do not get such good results. However, almost all patients with small cell cancer get some benefit from their treatment, being relieved of their symptoms and having their lives prolonged. One of the goals of lung cancer research is to improve the treatment so that all patients with this disease will be as lucky as Mr. Bryant.

CHAPTER 7

The Role of Nutrition in Lung Cancer

Many patients are surprised to learn that good nutrition is an important part of their medical care. A properly nourished patient, whose diet is high in protein and calories, is better able to withstand the stress of cancer and the side effects of its various treatments. In other words, good food is good medicine.

Well-nourished individuals can tolerate higher doses of chemotherapy and radiation therapy for longer periods of time. They recover from surgery faster, because a diet rich in nutrients helps rebuild the normal tissues that were affected. Also, the body's natural defenses against disease are strengthened by good nutrition.

Eating well also helps protect patients from complications. Some research even suggests that it raises a patient's resistance to tumor growth, although this is not yet certain.

If you find that, as a result of having lung cancer, your appetite is not as good as usual, you need to be especially sure that your body gets enough vitamins, minerals, protein, and calories. Protein and calories are particularly important because they build up your strength and prevent body tissues from breaking down.

It will help you to eat wisely if those who live with you understand the importance of good nutrition, and work with you in planning nutritious meals and snacks. One of the most useful things they can do is to learn techniques to help you cope with the problems of reduced appetite that affect many cancer patients so you can maintain your normal weight and control symptoms related to poor nutrition, such as weakness and weight loss.

Making Menu Plans

Dietitians recommend that you make out daily menu plans, especially at first. You may want to buy a calorie-counter booklet to be sure you are taking in enough calories. Some booklets also list the protein content of foods to help you select protein-rich foods.

Here are some general guidelines as to what you should eat each day for a balanced menu plan. You may or may not need vitamin pills. You should check with your doctor about this.

Dairy products. Two or more servings of milk or other dairy products. One serving = 1 cup of milk or yogurt, 1 1/2 ounces of cheese, 2 cups of cottage cheese, or 3/4 cup of ice cream.

Meats. Two or more 4-ounce servings of meat, fish, poultry, or eggs. Peanut butter, dried beans, peas, or nuts may be substituted.

Fruit. Two or more 1/2-cup servings. One should be a citrus fruit or juice.

Vegetables. Two or more 1/2-cup servings. One should be a dark green leafy or yellow vegetable.

Bread or cereal. Four or more servings. One serving = 1 slice of bread or 1 cup of cereal or 1/2 cup of pasta, rice, or grits.

Maintaining Your Weight

Most cancer patients lose weight because they do not eat as much food as their bodies need. Until recently, weight loss was thought to be an unavoidable side effect of lung cancer. This idea is no longer accepted. Losing weight is dangerous for people with lung cancer, just as it is for people with most other serious illnesses, because the body uses up its own stored fat, protein, and other nutrients, such as iron.

Like many others, you may have battled weight gain throughout your life. You may have viewed food as an indulgence. If so, you need to begin thinking of food as good medicine. If you have lost weight, you should try to eat moderate amounts of food several times during the day, in addition to mealtimes. You need to eat even if you are not hungry, because maintaining your weight and eating adequate amounts of nourishing foods are essential to your recovery and well-being.

Weight Loss and Appetite Loss

Losing weight can depress your appetite. When you lose fat, the body uses the fat it has stored for fuel and releases a substance that causes loss of appetite. That is why not eating —and losing weight—can set up a cycle of appetite loss and further weight loss.

Protein and Calorie Needs

You probably have been told to increase your intake of protein and calories. Protein is used by the body for tissue repair and growth. It is essential for lung cancer patients because it repairs tissues damaged by treatment. Calories are needed to keep your weight at its normal level or to help you gain back weight you have lost. If you have trouble eating enough for good nutrition and keeping your weight up, you should try to add high-calorie and high-protein foods to your diet.

If you don't have much of an appetite, you may wonder how you can increase the amount of protein in your diet without eating more food. Part of the answer is to eat high-protein foods such as cheese and eggs. Another approach is to follow certain food preparation hints that add protein to your meals in ways you'll hardly notice.

Commercial nutritional supplements can be a real help. Most of them come in milk-shake form and make good between-meal and bedtime snacks. If you are experiencing uncomfortable side effects of therapy in your mouth, throat, or digestive tract, you may want to use liquid nutritional supplements as total meal replacements until your sensitive tissues are back to normal.

You need extra calories in your diet not only to keep your weight up, but also to use as an energy source. If you don't take in enough calories, your body will use protein for basic energy needs. Then you won't have enough protein left for repairing body tissues. Even if you have always avoided high-fat foods such as mayonnaise and ice cream because they are fattening, you now need to accept them as good for you. In addition to providing calories, many of these previously forbidden foods will make other foods you eat tastier and more palatable.

How to Improve the Taste of High-Protein Foods

Try cold food. You may find that foods have better flavor when you eat them cold. The following are normally served cold or at room temperature: cheese, lunch meat, tuna salad (or ham or egg salad), deviled eggs, ice cream milk shakes, puddings, custards, and gelatin.

Enhance flavors. Add salt (if you are not on a salt-restricted diet) and more and stronger seasonings in cooking, such as mint, basil, oregano, or rosemary. Tart flavors such as orange juice, lemon juice, vinegar, and pickles may help (for those who have no problems with their mouths or throats).

Eat spicy or salty foods. You may enjoy cured meats such as bacon, ham, or sausage. Adding salt and spices to salads, casseroles, and main dishes may also make eating more appealing.

Marinate for flavor. You may find that meat, chicken, and fish taste better after they have been marinated in soy sauce, sweet fruit juices, wine, or Italian dressing.

Tips for Boosting Calories

If you have trouble eating enough to keep your weight up, try adding the following high-calorie foods to your diet (unless nausea and vomiting are a problem). Consider also adding high-calorie snacks such as nuts, cheese, and crackers.

Butter/margarine. Melt a teaspoonful of butter or margarine onto hot foods such as soups, vegetables, mashed potatoes, cooked cereal, rice, and soft-boiled eggs.

Cream. Use cream or whipped cream as a topping for hot chocolate, pudding, pie, gelatin, and other desserts.

Ice cream. Add ice cream to milk shakes and fruit desserts. Keep a variety of flavors in the freezer for snacks.

Mayonnaise. Use mayonnaise in meat salads, deviled eggs, and green salads. Combine with chopped meat, fish, chicken, or eggs for sandwich spreads.

Peanut butter. Spread peanut butter on banana or apple slices, stuff celery with it, or use it in sandwiches. If it's too dry, mix with mayonnaise or sour cream.

Sour cream. Serve sour cream on baked potatoes, mix into vegetables, use to make gravies and salad dressings. Mix with brown sugar and add to fruit for dessert.

Milk. Use whole milk, evaporated milk, and half-and-half (half cream, half milk) in preparing cereals, cocoa, canned soups, and puddings.

Tips for Adding Protein to Your Diet

If your appetite is poor, meats and other protein foods may taste peculiar to you. The following high-protein foods and food preparation points can increase the protein content of your diet while adding very little to the actual quantity of food consumed.

Fish/meat. Dice or grind beef, fish, and poultry and add to soups and casseroles.

Cheese. Add grated cheese (or small chunks) to sauces, casseroles, soups, or vegetables. Try melting sliced cheese over hot apple pie. Combine cottage cheese or cream cheese with fruit. Use cream cheese on bread or rolls.

Eggs. Blend finely chopped hard-boiled eggs into sauces, gravies, and salad dressings. You will hardly notice it. Make beverages and desserts containing eggs, such as custard, eggnog, and angel-food cake.

Skim milk powder. Add skim milk powder to fluid whole milk and chill well. Add skim milk powder to hot or cold cereals, scrambled eggs, soups, ground meat (for hamburgers, meatballs, or meatloaf), casseroles, sauces and gravies, cream sauces (for creamed meat, fish, or poultry), and to the ingredients for cakes and pies. Use in preparing cereals, cocoa, canned soups, and puddings.

Ice cream. Add extra ice cream to milk shakes.

Effects of Surgery on Nutrition

If you have had surgical treatment for your lung cancer, you may not be able to eat well for a few days. After that, you should be able to go back to your usual eating habits.

Your prompt recovery from surgery may depend on your nutritional condition before the operation. To ensure prompt recovery and to stimulate healing of the incision, it is sometimes necessary to have special nutritional treatment for a few days prior to surgery along with other pre-operative preparation.

Effects of Chemotherapy on Nutrition

Chemotherapy drugs kill the fast-growing cancer cells. But because the normal cells of the digestive tract also grow quickly, they are likely to be damaged by these drugs, resulting in a variety of symptoms that can make eating uncomfortable or even painful during and just after treatment.

Possible symptoms include changes in your sense of taste, mouth sores, sore throat, feelings of fullness, nausea, vomiting, and diarrhea. The symptoms will usually subside after a few days and then disappear, as the cells of the digestive tract quickly repair themselves. The rate at which you recover depends to some extent upon your following a well-balanced diet to repair the normal tissues that were damaged by the chemotherapy.

Effects of Radiotherapy on Nutrition

Because the radiation is aimed at specific places in the body, these are the only areas affected by the treatment. If your treatment happens to include any part of the digestive tract, you may have some bothersome symptoms.

For example, radiation to the mouth or neck areas may lower the flow of saliva, causing dry mouth. Or your sense of taste may be changed. Radiation to the chest usually affects the esophagus and makes swallowing difficult for a few days. Radiation to the stomach area can cause nausea and vomiting. If the intestines are radiated, diarrhea may become a problem.

These tissues of the body do recover, though, and symptoms generally go away. How rapidly the tissues repair themselves depends to a large extent on your following a nourishing diet, with enough calories and other nutrients.

Effects of the Tumor on Nutrition

The tumor itself may have a direct effect on eating. If it spreads to the point where it blocks the esophagus, for example, food may stick on the way down to the stomach and you may have difficulty swallowing your food.

Some scientists think that certain types of lung cancers give off a chemical that affects the part of the brain that tells you when you are hungry and when you are full. Therefore, you may think that you are full, that your body doesn't want food, when actually your stomach is empty and you need to eat.

You may notice changes in your sense of taste. There is a theory that some lung cancers have a chemical effect on certain minerals circulating in the bloodstream. These minerals affect taste, and when they are acted upon, food begins to taste different, and often peculiar.

Bitter foods may taste stronger than usual and unpleasant. Sweet foods may be harder to taste. However, taste never completely goes away. Any time you can make your food taste better, it will help your appetite.

If your sense of taste is affected, you may find that foods high in protein taste bitter. Do not avoid them, because protein is necessary to keep up your general health.

Other Deterrents to Good Nutrition

When cancer patients come in for a checkup, they sometimes say, "But I can't eat. Nothing looks good." How each person's body reacts to cancer and its treatments is highly individual, and not everyone has symptoms that interfere with eating properly. But even when symptoms themselves don't take away your desire to eat, your moods may have a greater than usual affect on your appetite. Knowing the importance of good eating will help you make the extra effort required to overcome these problems.

Nausea, Vomiting, and Feelings of Fullness

If feelings of fullness or nausea and vomiting are a problem, you need to eat foods that travel through the stomach quickly. Examples are milk shakes, gelatin, puddings, and iced desserts. Some patients find that they can relieve the nausea by eating small amounts of starchy foods (such as crackers or toast) at frequent intervals, or drinking cold drinks such as lemonade or carbonated drinks.

Avoid fatty and fried foods, since they take longer to digest. To help food leave the stomach as rapidly as possible, you should drink no liquids during meals. Instead, you can have something to drink an hour before eating and an hour after.

You should eat your food slowly and chew it well. Activity after eating tends to slow down digestion; it is better to rest or nap. After an hour's rest, most of the food should have passed from your stomach into the intestines.

If the smell of food cooking makes you feel nauseated, stay away from the kitchen during meal preparation. If the nausea is so bad that you have trouble keeping food down, your doctor may prescribe some medicine to relieve the problem.

Sore Throat, Dry or Sore Mouth

If you have chemotherapy to kill your tumor, you may get a dry or sore mouth and a sore throat for a few days afterward. You can minimize this problem by eating soft foods or drinking a liquid diet. If you are not nauseated you can use butter, gravy, and sauces to moisten food.

The following foods are soft in texture, high in protein, and rich in calories:

Baby or pureed foods	Ice cream
Chocolate milk	Macaroni and cheese
Cheesecake	Malted milk
Cocoa	Meat or fish salad
Cottage cheese (4% milkfat)	Milk shakes
Cream soups	Commercial nutritional supplements
Custard	Omelets
Eggnog	Puddings
Egg salad	Sherbet
Eggs, soft-cooked	Souffles
Gelatin salads	
Hot cereal with milk or cream	

Cramps and Diarrhea

Though the problem of cramps and diarrhea after radiation therapy is temporary, it can interfere with your getting the daily food requirements you need.

The following tips may help alleviate the problem somewhat:

Have no liquids at mealtimes; instead drink beverages between meals.

Instead of three meals a day, eat smaller portions of food more often.

Eat slowly, and try to eat in a relaxed atmosphere.

Avoid foods prepared with sugar.

Avoid foods that can produce gas, such as carbonated drinks, beer, beans, cabbage, highly spiced foods, and too many sweets. Also avoid chewing gum.

If possible, do not skip meals, and avoid talking while you are chewing. Both of these contribute to gas.

Keep down the roughage in your diet. Roughage is the material in food that humans cannot digest. Foods that are high in roughage include raw fruits and vegetables, whole grain cereals and breads, popcorn, and nuts. Roughage helps prevent constipation and contributes to regular, softer stools. But when your intestines are irritated, normal levels of roughage in the diet may be too much.

If you have diarrhea, large amounts of the mineral potassium may be lost from the body. Your doctor may prescribe potassium tablets or direct you to eat foods high in potassium, such as bananas, red meat, salt-water fish, potatoes, and mushrooms.

If cramping and diarrhea continue to be a problem, ask your doctor for medicine to relieve you.

Constipation

Constipation frequently results from pain medication and sometimes results from anti-cancer drugs. If you find that you need a laxative, eat foods high in roughage or drink prune juice. If raw fruits and vegetables are hard for you to chew, try grating them. Drink lots of liquids. Get as much light exercise as you comfortably can. Your doctor may prescribe medication, as well.

Depression

The feelings and emotions that follow the diagnosis of cancer can take away your appetite. Even though you know that eating is important for your general health, there may be times when it just seems too difficult. At times, good nutrition may seem like the least of your problems.

It will help if you do not get unduly upset when you cannot follow nutritional guidelines precisely, because upset feelings will only decrease your appetite more. Accept the fact that there are days when you cannot eat as much as you think you should. Then, on the days when your appetite is back, try to catch up a little.

Don't let others push or prod you into eating. But if they do, try not to let feelings of stubbornness keep you from eating, or their good intentions could create the opposite of the intended effect. On the other hand, if you find that gentle encouragement helps, let the people around you know. Eat more when you're hungry, most often at breakfast. Eat small amounts of food frequently rather than three full meals a day.

Finally, try motivating yourself to eat by reminding yourself of the importance of good nutrition to your health.

Food is medicine for the person with lung cancer. You must eat. If you cannot eat for pleasure, you need to eat because you know that your body requires the proteins, vitamins, and calories.

Many hospitals have full-time dietitians on the staff who help patients figure out what they should eat and how it should be prepared, as well as giving them guidelines for getting to the right weight and maintaining it. Check with your doctor to see if a dietitian is available to advise you.

One of your doctor's prime concerns is that you maintain your general health as much as possible. If you fail to keep up your strength by taking in the right nutrients, your disease is more apt to wear you down. On the positive side, good nutrition helps protect you from complications. Some research even suggests that it can raises your resistance to tumor growth, although this is not yet certain.

CHAPTER 8

Coping with the Stresses of Lung Cancer

Once you have been given the diagnosis of lung cancer, you will be faced with concerns and stresses you did not have before. Questions about your physical condition, your longevity, and your family will become a new focal point, and your life will now center around these issues.

During this time, it will be important to keep in close communication with your doctor and other health professionals. Even if your lung cancer has not been cured by the treatment methods discussed in earlier chapters, your physician and other health care personnel will continue to offer you the best care that medicine has to offer.

You will need to rely on your family for their emotional support and the practical kinds of help they can give you. Even other people with cancer can be a source of support.

The Control of Pain

One of the greatest fears of cancer patients is pain. The fear alone can create tension, which can make other problems seem greater.

Pain is *not* an inevitable consequence of the disease. In fact, many patients with lung cancer experience *no pain at all.* If there is pain, it may be only mild. It may come and go. Often aspirin or other simple analgesics are enough to control the discomfort.

If you should have stronger pain, however, a large number of medicines are available to relieve it. They range in strength from codeine to morphine. If you need a stronger medicine than the one you are taking, it will be prescribed. You do not need to fear suffering unduly from pain.

You also do not have to worry about addiction to the stronger pain killers. The likelihood of this problem is extremely minimal since the doctor will know what kind of drug you take, how much, and how often.

If you have pain that persists over a long period of time, your doctor has ways of putting an end to it. One is a simple operation to cut the nerve carrying the pain sensation to the brain. The operation should not affect the function of nearby muscles or organs. The injection of a drug into that nerve can also block the nerve impulses. Again, deadening a nerve with a drug just makes the area numb but does not affect the function of the muscles.

Many people fear pain because they worry that it is a sign that the cancer is spreading. It is natural to link every discomfort with the disease, but most people do have a variety of aches and pains that come and go; this is especially true of those in the age group prone to develop lung cancer.

The best plan is to check with your physician when some new, persistent pain arises. It may be due to another condition, such as arthritis. In any case, it can be treated.

Treatment of Other Medical Problems

Lung Conditions

Most patients with lung cancer have other lung problems, such as chronic bronchitis and emphysema. These conditions, along with the cancer, may then make the patient susceptible to lung infections. If you have one of these conditions, it will be treated along with the lung cancer.

If you are having trouble breathing, the doctor may prescribe a medicine that helps open up your breathing tubes. Or you may get a medication called an expectorant to make it easier for you to cough up the mucus in your lungs that can plug up some of the breathing passages. If you have an infection, the doctor may prescribe an antibiotic. If you have shortness of breath that becomes extremely troublesome, the doctor can see that you get oxygen.

Other Medical Problems

Influenza (the flu) can have serious consequences for a person with lung cancer. You should take an appropriate flu shot every fall.

Your peace of mind may depend upon the knowledge that your doctor will treat you as a total person and not just a case of lung cancer. People who have lung cancer are usually middle-aged and older, a time of life when other medical conditions tend to arise. You need to know that you can bring all of your physical and mental concerns to your doctor's attention. If you have a heart condition, arthritis, or just a common cold, you can be sure of having whatever treatment you need.

Emotional Reactions

A diagnosis of lung cancer is likely to lead to a number of emotional reactions. The first reaction of both the patient and the family is usually shock, followed immediately by disbelief. Disbelief serves to cushion the mind against something too painful to accept.

Other common reactions are denial and anger. Denial is a kind of looking away emotionally. Some doctors believe that temporary denial helps tide you and your family over this initial period of emotional pain. If you say to yourself, "This just can't be happening to me," you may be giving yourself time to face the truth gradually, rather than all at once. If you feel angry, your anger may have a number of targets—your doctors, the hospital, yourself, even God.

It is easy to understand how most people with lung cancer are frustrated and angry at what seems like an unjust fate. "Why me?" is the question repeated over and over by cancer patients. It reflects a profound frustration and feeling of helplessness in the face of the disease. In time, it passes for most people. You may need time to go through your feelings of shock, disbelief, denial, and anger before you can go on to accept the disease and live with it.

Two other common reactions to the diagnosis of lung cancer are anxiety and depression. Anxiety is an uneasy state of mind associated with worry and fear. Depression involves profound feelings of sadness, gloom, and discouragement. Anxiety and depression are usually unavoidable and tend to come and go.

Ways to Lessen Anxiety and Depression

Anxiety or depression can make any pain or discomfort you have much worse. It can even create symptoms that have nothing to do with your disease. A person who is depressed often becomes quiet and withdrawn, keeping feelings to him- or herself.

Look for Causes

Try to discover exactly what is causing your anxiety and/or depression. It may be the fact of just having this dread disease. You may worry that others will avoid you. Or you may have unexplainable feelings of guilt, loss of control, or even revulsion toward yourself. In many cases, isolating the problem will help you to deal with it and perhaps even find a solution.

Understanding what is going on medically can relieve some of your uneasiness. Keep a list of all your questions and concerns and ask your doctor for a thorough explanation.

Hand in hand with having cancer are many other concerns that can cause as much distress and worry as the disease itself. Try to identify all the unknowns that you may have to face. For instance, if you are the main wage-earner in your family, will you be able to return to work? If not, how will your family maintain itself financially? If you have children at home, who will take care of them when you and your spouse are away for doctors' appointments or medical treatments? How should your family handle the situation if you are not doing well and require more medical and nursing care?

When you have arrived at solutions for all of your potential problems, you will be less uneasy.

Discuss Feelings

Try to deal with troublesome issues and anxieties with your family as they come up. Many of these may be painful and hard to talk about, but it is better to discuss them openly and honestly, rather than allowing them to build and grow inside you.

Eventually, as feelings are shared, the pain is lessened. Family members will also experience the joy of establishing a closer relationship with you. Frequently, what is bothering one person is bothering the others in the family, too. Usually everyone is relieved when the problem is finally brought out in the open for discussion.

Talk with other people, too. It may help to join a support group of patients who have cancer. It is a great help to find that other people care about and understand some of your emotional pain.

Stay Active

Just because you have been told that you have cancer is no reason to change your lifestyle. Try to live in the present, day by day, enjoying life as much as possible and sharing it with others. There is no need to stop activities you enjoyed in the past. Seeing other people and maintaining some sort of social life is important.

In general, anything you feel well enough to do is all right. This includes everything from light activity, to sports (like golf), to an active sexual life. If you are able to continue working full- or part-time, this should help. If you are unable to work, it is important that you get your family's cooperation in helping you to keep occupied. Stay involved in as many activities as possible.

Get Spiritual Help

Many families find strength in developing the spiritual side of their lives. For some, this means establishing closer ties with their church and getting pastoral counseling. For others, it may mean a closer communion with nature, a renewed interest in music, art, and books, or even the enjoyment of children. You can gain spiritual strength by taking a fresh look at the bonds within your family and by encouraging family members to join together, share, and support one another.

Get Counseling

Some families cannot handle the emotional strain of cancer on their own; they have trouble expressing their problems openly with each other and with the doctor. Many people need help from a trained counselor.

If you, your spouse, or any members of your family find the stresses that go with lung cancer too hard to cope with, you should ask your doctor to direct you to professional counseling. A counselor can help you and your family come to terms with what it means to be faced with cancer and with the concerns and anxieties that cancer can create.

Find Out About Financial Assistance

As medical expenses mount, it is natural to worry about where the money will come from. By working to solve this problem, you may help lessen feelings of anxiety and/or depression. The following resources may be available for you to take advantage of.

Social services. Most large hospitals and clinics employ social service workers who can help patients get financial aid or help them apply for payment of medical expenses from their private or group medical insurance.

Medicare. Medicare funds are available to many people over sixty-five years old, as well as to certain individuals under sixty-five. You can check into your eligibility for Medicare benefits by calling the nearest Social Security office. Most communities have an office listed in the telephone book under "United States Government."

Medicaid. Medicaid may help pay your medical bills if you are under sixty-five and meet the eligibility requirements in your county. To check on this, and to obtain information about other sources of help, call your county's Social Service Department. The telephone listing will appear under the name of the county.

Check into Other Kinds of Assistance

Your local unit of the American Cancer Society may be able to help you in a variety of ways, depending upon its resources. Some local units are better established and better staffed than others. One or more of the following may be available at your local unit:

Volunteers who can drive you to the doctor.

Hospital equipment you may borrow without charge, to use in your home.

Discussion groups for cancer patients and their families, to share mutual problems.

Your local unit may be able to direct you to other organizations that offer support, reassurance, and assistance to families in which a member has cancer. Check your telephone book under "American Cancer Society."

The National Cancer Institute in Bethesda, Maryland has a Cancer Information Service. You can call their toll-free number, 1-800-4-CANCER for information or just to talk. Staffers will take the time to listen to your questions or problems. This is especially helpful when your doctor isn't available or doesn't have the time. Calls made during business hours are automatically routed to the caller's region; calls made nights and weekends are answered in a central office in Washington, DC.

Tell Your Doctor When Feelings Become Too Much to Handle

Should feelings of anxiety or depression begin to feel overwhelming to you (or family members), the doctor may prescribe medicine to help you function better. You may need it for only a short time, perhaps just long enough to calm your nerves so that you can face the issues that are causing your anxiety or depression.

CHAPTER 9

Cancer Quackery

"Cancer quacks," using untested methods of treating cancer, prey upon the fears of cancer patients and their families. They take advantage of the natural anxiety about this illness and the common fears about conventional forms of treatment, such as surgery, radiotherapy, or chemotherapy. With never-failing optimism, cancer quacks promise cure or at least marked improvement by their methods.

Those who sell unproven cancer remedies are often well-meaning but medically untrained individuals who actually believe in their "cures." Or they may be money-seekers who know that cancer quackery is big business. The person or family gripped by the fear of cancer will often grasp at any straw and pay any price.

The great tragedy of this problem is that some people with cancer lose the chance to be cured because they postpone seeing a qualified physician until it is too late. Or they deprive themselves of a longer, more comfortable life by resorting to unproven remedies that may even be dangerous, rather than taking advantage of the numerous treatments that modern medicine has to offer. Some of the cancer quack's remedies may actually be dangerous.

The physician with training and experience can do much to prolong the lives of patients with cancer and to help them remain comfortable and active as long as possible. But patients who listen to the false promises of the cancer quack often pay a heavy price, both in terms of their pocketbooks and their health.

How to Recognize Cancer Quackery

The individuals and organizations that sell or advocate unproven methods of cancer treatment tend to have a number of things in common. Although a few are misguided professionals (such as M.D.s or Ph.D.s) practicing outside their fields of training with treatment methods that have not had adequate scientific testing, most of them have unusual academic degrees, such as Ph.N. (Philosopher of Naturopathy) or MsD (Doctor of Metaphysics).

Frequently, the advocate of an unproven treatment method is also a nutrition faddist, and an unusual diet is prescribed as part of the treatment. For example, the "grape cure" requires that the patient's diet consist solely of grapes or grape juice for a week or two. Another recommends large quantities of carrot juice.

The "scientists" who advocate unproven cancer remedies usually operate outside established medical organizations. In fact, they usually claim that the medical establishment is against them. They claim to be advanced scientific thinkers —individuals ahead of their time. The language of cancer quacks is often persuasive because it combines a righteous stance with complicated and technical-sounding words.

If they keep records, they do not allow them to be examined by a reputable doctor. Nor are they likely to allow a reputable doctor to be a consultant. Frequently, the formulas for their drugs are kept secret.

Unlike reputable doctors, they do not publish articles about their "cures" in scientific journals or report their findings at medical meetings. They are more likely to write for sensational or health magazines that are sold to the lay public, or publications that specialize in unproven or nonmedical approaches to the treatment of disease. In all their writings, the authors will claim that special diets or nutrients can cure cancer, but they will offer no scientific basis for these claims.

The Appeal of Cancer Quackery

The quack who offers total reassurance and unqualified promises often has the edge over reputable physicians who are usually cautious, prescribing treatment only after diagnostic tests and careful consultation with their colleagues.

In the emotionally charged atmosphere of a frightened patient and family, the cancer quack's offer of a miracle treatment is very appealing.

Quacks are quick to cite examples of patients they have "cured." They may advertise "before" and "after" pictures of their patients, sometimes using testimonials from prominent people. Several famous actors, actresses, and public officials have been persuaded of the worth of Krebiozen, for example, and have become active, vocal supporters of this treatment, even though scientific studies have shown it to be worthless.

Ironically, many patients who resort to unproven cancer remedies have already been cured by conventional medical treatment. But in their fear that the cancer has not been totally eradicated, they continue to seek out additional treatment in the form of an unproven drug (such as Laetrile) or a bizarre diet (such as no protein before noon each day). When the cancer does not recur, they give the unproven method the credit. Some patients are "cured" who never had cancer in the first place, but had another condition that would have disappeared with or without treatment.

The "Evidence"

Numerous books have appeared in recent years that skillfully present the case against conventional medical treatment and the case for "cancer cures." Their authors are clever at interweaving scientific fact with scientific fiction. They appear to present the pros and cons of various cancer cures and persuade the reader that the information is impartial, even though it is not. The books are able to subtly lead the reader to the conclusions the authors wish. It is amazing how a "cancer cure" practitioner, who lacks the years of medical training and experience necessary to make judgments about the treatment of a disease as complex as cancer, can convince the reader that the necessary knowledge can be condensed into a single paperback book.

Many journalists have added to the controversy surrounding unproven cancer remedies by writing stories about cancer "cures." These articles have great public appeal, even if they sometimes smack of sensationalism and actually mislead readers. Although most of us tend to believe that what we read in newspapers and magazines is factual, it is important to remember that writers are not scientists, and that some of them may be easily misled by false information.

Why You Should Avoid Unproven Treatments Touted as Sure Cures

There is nothing inherently bad about an unproven method of cancer management. All types of cancer treatment were unproven when first used. What is bad is when an unproven treatment is advertised as a cure and used on a widespread basis without first undergoing careful scientific study. Before large numbers of patients are given a drug or undergo any kind of treatment, reputable physicians want to be sure that the drug or the procedure is safe and effective.

What established medicine has to offer often seems vague and threatening in contrast to the promises of the cancer cure quack. Surgery, radiotherapy, and chemotherapy can seem like difficult alternatives to a simple "sure cure." Yet, the unproven cure that seems like the easiest way at first can later turn into a nightmare. It could shorten your life by depriving you of medically sound treatment, or it could even deprive you of the chance to be really cured.

CHAPTER 10

Prospects for the Future

Lung cancer is the most common cause of cancer death in men, claiming more lives than the next four most common cancers combined. In women, lung cancer has recently surpassed breast cancer as the prime cause of cancer death. The hope for the future is that medical research will be able to reduce the threat of this disease. Scientists are working on many fronts to find out more about ways of preventing lung cancer, more sensitive methods for early detection, and more effective forms of treatment.

Prevention

Most lung cancer could be prevented. Various approaches to prevention are necessary, however, because lung cancer has several causes.

Smoking

About eight out of ten cases of lung cancer are caused by smoking of cigarettes and other tobacco products. The percent of men who smoke has decreased a great deal, and as a result we have been seeing fewer cases of lung cancer in young and middle-aged men. More recently, the number of women who smoke has declined, too. In the future, we expect their incidence of lung cancer to decline as well.

The tar in tobacco seems to be the main culprit. Because the average tar content of cigarettes has been reduced markedly in the last twenty years, and may be reduced further, we are hopeful that smoking will cause fewer cases of lung cancer in the future. However, there is no reason to believe that there will ever be a safe cigarette.

An even more important preventive measure is to keep people from smoking in the first place and to help smokers quit. The National Cancer Institute, the American Cancer Society, and other organizations have undertaken national programs of public education to alert Americans to the dangers of smoking and to help them stop.

Passive Smoking and Air Pollution

Some people who have never smoked develop lung cancer. There are several possible sources for the disease, and in each case efforts are being made to eliminate them. One is second-hand smoke in the indoor air, leading to "passive smoking." Efforts to reduce this kind of air pollution, such as passing no-smoking ordinances and establishing no-smoking sections in restaurants, may eventually prevent some cases of lung cancer.

Another factor is the exposure of workers to carcinogens in the workplace. Efforts are being made to protect Americans from cancer-causing industrial chemicals, such as asbestos, uranium, arsenic, chromium, lead oxide, and iron oxide. Health professionals, leaders from industry, and the public are finding that they must work together more than they have in the past to control the use of these substances.

General pollution of the outdoor air in some large crowded cities may also be a cause of some lung cancer. Cleaning up the air may prevent some lung cancers.

As we discover other specific carcinogens for lung cancer, we must insist that they be controlled. For example, there is already some evidence that marijuana smoke might cause lung cancer, and we must urge people to avoid this danger.

Dietary Influences

More and more data are being accumulated which show that a diet low in vitamin A makes smokers more apt to get lung cancer. This vitamin is found in dark-green leafy vegetables, such as spinach and broccoli, and dark-yellow and orange vegetables and fruit, such as carrots, peaches, and apricots. Soon we may be able to recommend foods that will reduce the risk of getting lung cancer.

Many scientists are studying the value of some vitamin A compounds. It may be possible in the future to prescribe such a medicine, more complex than a vitamin pill, to reduce the risk of getting lung cancer.

The Search for Earlier Methods of Detection

If lung cancer could be detected in its earliest stages, cure would almost always be possible. Some studies are now underway to develop more sensitive diagnostic tests that can be performed easily, accurately, and inexpensively on large numbers of people.

The value of routine chest X-rays for healthy people who are known to have a high risk of developing lung cancer, such as smokers over the age of forty, is also being studied.

Although some of the tests have met with limited success, none of them has been proven to be of enough value to be used routinely. A test that has sometimes helped in early diagnosis is the sputum examination. An individual is asked to cough up some sputum, which is examined under a microscope for the presence of cancer cells that have been shed from the inner lining of the breathing passages.

Researchers have been looking for substances in the blood that might reveal the presence of cancer cells in the lung. They have been encouraged by the finding of many different chemicals, including some hormones, in the bloodstreams of some patients. One that has been studied extensively is called *carcinoembryonic antigen*, or *CEA*.

Improved Treatment

Surgery, radiotherapy, and chemotherapy individually or some combinations of them are the standard method of treating lung cancer. Numerous research projects have the objective of improving each of these or learning how to better combine them.

Surgery

Surgical treatment of lung cancer continues to become safer and more effective. Surgeons are learning to be more selective in determining whether or not to operate, and they are learning to avoid futile operations by determining the extent of the cancer more accurately and by assessing the ability of the patient to survive the operation. They are also learning how to remove cancers successfully that in the past were thought to be inoperable. They now know how to provide better care for patients during the critical postoperative period to reduce the complications of major surgery and thereby reduce its risk.

Radiotherapy

More powerful X-ray machines are being developed that deliver the maximum dose of radiation to the cancer with the least possible damage to the normal body tissues.

X-ray therapy experts are also testing a variety of treatment schedules (from one treatment once a week to one treatment twice a day) to learn which program is most effective and at the same time more convenient for the patient.

Some experimental drugs called radiosensitizers are being tested to see whether they increase the effectiveness of radiation in killing the cancer. Some researchers are injecting radioactive materials into the cancer itself to direct large amounts of radiation to the cancer, but a minimum amount to normal tissues. As more is learned about the benefits of each of these techniques, we can expect radiotherapy to become more effective and more convenient, and to cause fewer undesirable side effects.

Chemotherapy

We are optimistic that someday soon chemotherapy for lung cancer will be more effective and safer. Many drugs have been discovered that seem to have some value; however, scientists will continue searching until they find more powerful drugs that have fewer side effects. In the meantime, they are researching how to combine the presently available drugs into the most effective combinations with the fewest toxic effects.

Other researchers are studying how often and how long to give each drug, as well as when to give it. There is some evidence suggesting that the time of day or night that chemotherapy is given may affect the efficacy or the toxicity, or both.

Combination Therapy

In the future it should be possible to cure more patients by combining two or even all three methods of therapy, in a sequence tailored for each individual. Although surgery will probably continue to be the best available treatment, surgeons cannot always remove all the cancer. Thus researchers are trying to improve the cure rate by testing whether radiation therapy or chemotherapy, or both, works better when given before or after surgery. In other studies, various combinations of radiation therapy and chemotherapy are given to patients whose cancers are inoperable.

What is best for each patient and each type of cancer will be known only after many years of painstaking treatment-planning, record-keeping, and evaluation of the long-term effects. As the research goes on, doctors and scientists from various institutes continue to compare their results. Patients with lung cancer, as well as those with other types of cancer, are already reaping some of the benefits of this work.

New Treatments

Immunotherapy

The body's immune system is powerful and is acutely sensitive to foreign intruders. In the normal person, the immune system is always on the alert for danger signs of foreign cells in the blood. It destroys them when suspicious signs arise. Since cancer cells are foreign intruders, one would think that the immune system could cure cancer by destroying the cancer cells.

Unfortunately, the body's defense against cancer cells seems less effective than its defense against other foreign cells such as viruses or bacteria. Even though we know from research that our bodies can tell the difference between cancer cells and normal cells, cancer cells are not as clearly "foreign" as viruses or bacteria. Cancer cells tend to resemble the organs in which they begin growing, and they have many of the characteristic of normal body cells.

Once cancer cells have escaped detection and have formed a tumor, the cancer seems to overwhelm the immune system with malignant cells.

In addition, a great deal of experimental and clinical evidence suggests than when cancer is present and growing, the body's immune defenses are not up to par. For example, scientists have been able to stimulate the development and growth of experimental cancer in animals by impairing the animals' immunity. Patients with growing tumors show abnormally low numbers of lymphocytes, the blood cells that fight germs. Research has also shown that people with weak immune systems, and those who must take medicines that lower immunity, are more likely to get cancer than other individuals.

These bits of evidence point to immunology as a key to some of the remaining mystery of cancer. Some immunologists think that a therapeutic breakthrough for cancer will take the form of a general stimulation of the body's defense system to prevent or overcome the cancer. In some experiments on animals, cancers have been controlled or destroyed by stimulating the animals' immunologic defenses.

There is some evidence that the same is true for humans. For example, a few well-documented cases have been reported in medical journals of patients who had definite, clearly diagnosed cancers that simply shrank and disappeared, without any kind of treatment. This is called "spontaneous tumor regression," and it has been found to occur after an infection has probably stimulated the patient's immune defenses. The most likely explanation of this riddle is that the balance of power in the immune system shifted from the cancer to the immune defenses, and the defenses won.

Although some kinds of immunotherapy have shown promise in certain types of cancer, all the evidence is not yet in. Because of the complexity of lung cancer and the fact that "lung cancer" really covers several different types of cancer, much experimental work for this illness remains to be done. Many studies are being carried out, and only time will tell if any of the following approaches will be of value.

BCG Vaccine

BCG stands for "bacillus of Calmette and Guerin" (named for the two French scientists who discovered it) and is related to the germ that causes tuberculosis. When injected into the body as a vaccine, BCG has been shown to help the body fight some types of cancer. It activates the immune system to manufacture germ-killing substances that are also cancer-killing. Even when BCG is not powerful enough to rid the body of all traces of cancer, it often controls the growth of the tumor and slows down its rate of spread.

So far, BCG has not been proved to be of value in the treatment of lung cancer.

Interferons

Interferons are substances that have shown some promise in the treatment of cancer. The body's immune system manufactures tiny amounts of these powerful substances to help fight certain diseases, and cancer may be one of them. There is research evidence to suggest that interferons may be effective against a number of kinds of cancer, but to date lung cancer has not been among them.

Interferons are extracted in small amounts from large quantities of human blood and are therefore difficult and expensive to obtain. As newer, more practical methods of producing interferons in larger quantities are developed, more studies of this as a treatment for lung cancer will be possible.

Monoclonal Antibodies

Monoclonal antibodies are laboratory-made substances developed by immunologists in the mid-1970s. They work by attaching themselves to cancer cells, thereby marking the cells for attack by the body's immune system. Some of the monoclonal antibodies may also be able to carry cancer-killing substances. Studies are still in the experimental stages, but show significant promise as researchers continue to work to refine these synthetic antibodies for use in cancer treatment.

Transfer Factor

Transfer factor is a substance in the blood which, theoretically, can transfer immunity to a certain disease from one person to another. By giving a cancer patient the transfer factor from another person whose immunologic defense system has already mounted an attack against the same kind of cancer, scientists hope to succeed in killing cancer cells in the patient.

Hyperthermia

Hyperthermia, or heat treatment, involves applying heat to tumors. Scientists have known for many years that high temperatures can kill some cancer cells while not affecting the normal cells of the body. And doctors have been aware for many years that some patients with cancer improve after having an infection that causes a high fever.

Several techniques are being studied. One uses ultrasound waves to heat the area of the body containing the tumor. Another uses radio-frequency waves sent through needles inserted into the tumor. A third method is to warm the patient's blood using a bypass technique in which blood runs from an artery into a catheter that passes through a heating machine, and then returns to the patient's circulation through a vein.

These techniques, which can be used alone or in combination with radiotherapy or chemotherapy, are being studied in only a few cancer centers in the country. Whether any type of hyperthermia will be of real value in the treatment of lung cancer remains to be proved.

Laser Treatment

A laser beam can be thought of as a beam of light that is projected onto a tumor and may destroy the cancer cells. The word "laser" is an acronym for "light amplification by stimulated emission of radiation." There are several kinds of lasers. The one that is being used experimentally to treat some patients with lung cancer is called the YAG laser. ("YAG" stands for "yttrium-aluminum-garnet.")

A laser beam penetrates a very short distance into a tumor mass, destroying the cancer cells on or near the surface of the tumor. It can't go through a large mass of tissue cells the way an X-ray does, so it can't be projected onto a tumor in the middle of the lung. However, the laser beam may be transmitted through a special bronchoscope and projected directly onto a lung cancer in the windpipe or one of the major bronchi. Thus it may be of value in treating some tumors that are blocking a breathing tube when X-ray therapy has not been effective.

In some studies, a tumor has been made more sensitive to the laser beam after the patient has been given an intravenous injection of a chemical called *hematoporphyrin derivative*, which is concentrated in cancer cells. This treatment has been reported to be of help to patients who have recurrent cancer blocking one of the breathing tubes.

Lung Transplants

Since heart transplants and kidney transplants are successful, many patients ask about having a lung transplant. Numerous experiments have been done on animals and a few attempts have been made to transplant lungs in humans, largely without success. The human body will not adapt to another person's lung the way it will to a heart or kidney. Apparently the immune system recognizes a lung as "foreign" and soon rejects it, with the result that the rejected tissue breaks down and dies. It is doubtful that lung transplantation will ever be applicable to the treatment of lung cancer.

Artificial Lungs

Artificial lungs are already used during open-heart surgery, when the body's own heart-lung system must be bypassed for a few critical hours of surgical work. However, scientists are having difficulty in developing an artificial lung that can be used outside the operating room.

There are still a great number of technical problems to be overcome, such as the requirement that the apparatus be portable so it can be carried by the patient. Unlike the artificial kidney machine, which has worked well because the patient can come to a dialysis center to be connected to it once or twice a week, an effective artificial lung would require it to be attached to the patient twenty-four hours a day. While scientists may be able to accomplish this eventually, the technology will probably take years to develop.

Glossary

- A -

abscess *(ab'-sess)*: a collection of pus in an area of the body, usually caused by infection.

acute *(uh-kewt')*: coming on suddenly.

adenocarcinoma *(a'-den-oh-kahr-sin-oh'-muh)*: type of lung cancer; when examined under the microscope, the cells resemble glandular cells.

adjuvant therapy *(ad'-jew-vant thair-uh-pee)*: something (such as a kind of treatment) that enhances the effectiveness of medical treatment.

Adriacil *(ay'-dree-uh-sil)*: trade name for fluorouracil.

Adriamycin *(ay-dree-uh-my'-sin)*: trade name for doxorubin.

alveoli *(al-vee'-oh-lie)*: in the lung, tiny air sacs found at the ends of the smallest branches of the bronchial tree, where oxygen passes into the bloodstream and carbon dioxide passes into the lungs to be exhaled.

alveolus: singular of alveoli.

anesthesia *(an-uss-thee'-zhia)*: loss of feeling of pain.

anxiety *(ang-zy'-uh-tee)*: state of general uneasiness, worry, or fear.

- B -

BCG: a vaccine made from living organisms related to tuberculosis germs; when injected into the body, it stimulates the immune defense system.

benign *(buh-nine')*: not malignant; noncancerous.

biopsy *(by'-op-see)*: procedure in which a small sample of tissue or fluid is removed from the body and examined under a microscope to determine whether cancer or other disease is present.

bone marrow: the inner, spongy core of bone that produces blood cells.

bone scan: an examination of the bones, using a radioactive chemical, to to determine whether cancer is present.

bronchial carcinoma *(brahn'-kee-ul kar-sin-oh'-muh)*: lung cancer.

bronchi: plural of bronchus; bronchial tubes.

bronchioles *(brahn'-kee-ohlz)*: the smallest branches of the breathing tree, which carry air to the alveoli.

bronchodilator *(brahn-koh-dy'-lay-tor)*: a medicine, usually sprayed into the throat; used to help open up the breathing passages.

bronchogenic carcinoma *(brahn-koh-jen'-ik kahr-sin-oh'-muh):* lung cancer.

bronchoscope *(brahn'-koh-skope)*: a slender tubular viewing instrument inserted into the throat and the larger breathing passages, to examine them for the presence of cancer.

bronchoscopy *(brahn-kah'-skoh-pee)*: examination of the breathing passages with a bronchoscope for the presence of cancer or other disease.

bronchus *(brahn'-kus)*: either of the two main breathing tubes branching off from the windpipe; one bronchus leads to each lung.

- C -

cancer: uncontrolled growth of abnormal cells; may spread throughout the body.

capillary *(ka'-pill-air-ee)*: smallest of the body's blood vessels.

catheter *(ka'-thuh-tur)*: a flexible plastic tube that may inserted into the body; used to deliver fluids to the bloodstream or drain fluids that have collected in the body.

CAT scan *(cat skan)*: a diagnostic technique using pictures of the body.

CAT scanner *(cat skan'-ur)*: a medical instrument using X-rays and a computer to give pictures of internal body structures.

chemotherapist *(kee-moh-thair'-uh-pist)*: a physician who specializes in the medical treatment of cancer, especially in the administration of anticancer drugs; also called a medical oncologist.

chemotherapy *(kee-moh-thair'-uh-pee)*: the use of drugs to kill or slow the growth of cancer cells.

chest X-ray: photograph of the inner structures of the chest, obtained by use of X-rays (patient is exposed to very low levels of radiation); different from X-ray therapy, in which large amounts of radiation are used to kill cancer cells.

chronic (krah'-nik): lasting a long time.

cilia *(sil'-ee-uh)*: tiny hair-like projections on the surface of the bronchi that continually sweep mucus up and out of the lungs, helping to cleanse them.

cisplatin *(sis-pla'-tin)*: a chemotherapy drug; given intravenously.

cisplatinum: cisplatin.

clotting: the clumping together of blood cells to slow or stop the flow of blood.

cobalt *(koh'-bawlt)*: a metal that can be made radioactive to produce gamma rays, similar to X-rays, that are capable of destroying tumor tissue.

cobalt unit: a radiotherapy machine containing radioactive cobalt.
codeine *(koh'-deen)*: a pain medicine, stronger than aspirin.
collarbone: bone situated on each side of the neck, extending from the base of the neck in front to the shoulder joint.
complications: unexpected symptoms or problems resulting from a medical treatment, such as surgery or drugs.
constipation *(kahn-stih-pay'-shun)*: abnormally delayed or infrequent passage of dry, hardened stools.
CT scan: see CAT scan.
cyclophosphamide *(si-kloh-fahs'-fuh-mide)*: a chemotherapy drug, given intravenously or, rarely, by mouth.
cytology *(si-tah'-loh-gee)*: branch of biology dealing with structure and function of animal and plant cells.
Cytoxan *(si-tox'-an)*: trade name for cyclophosphamide.

- D -

DDP: trade name for cisplatin.
depression *(dee-preh'-shun)*: feelings of sadness, gloominess, and discouragement.
diaphragm *(die'-uh-fram)*: sheet of muscle just below the base of the lungs that contracts as air is pulled into the lungs.
diarrhea *(die-uh-ree'-uh)*: an upset of the intestines causing food to be propelled too rapidly through the digestive tract, resulting in loose, frequent stools.
digestive tract: the food canal, which consists of the mouth, throat, stomach, and small intestines, and the rectum.
doxorubin *(dox-oh-rue'-bin)*: a chemotherapy drug, given intravenously.

- E -

Efudex *(eh'-few-dex)*: trade name for fluorouracil.

emphysema *(em-fih-zee'-muh)*: condition that results in overexpansion of the air spaces in the lung, taking away their elasticity and ability to function normally.

epidermoid carcinoma *(eh-pih-dur'-moyd kahr-sin-oh'-muh)*: type of lung cancer in which cells resemble skin cells; also called squamous (skway'-mus) cell carcinoma.

esophagus *(eh-sah'-fuh-gus)*: the "swallowing tube."

etoposide *(eh-tah'-poh-side)*: a chemotherapy drug, given intravenously.

expectorant *(eks-pek'-toh-runt)*: type of medicine that helps a person cough up secretions from the lungs.

- F -

fiberoptic bronchoscope *(fi-bur-op'-tik brahn'-koh-skope)*: instrument consisting of a flexible bundle of glass fibers that transmit light throughout their length; allows better view of breathing passages than a conventional bronchoscope.

5-FU: trade name for fluorouracil.

fluoroscope: an instrument used for observing the internal structure of opaque organs in the body, by means of X-rays.

fluoroscopy *(flew-rah'-skoh-pee)*: X-ray examination using a fluoroscope.

fluorouracil *(flew-roh-yew'-rah-sill)*: chemotherapy drug, given intravenously. Also called 5-fluorouracil.

Food and Drug Administration (FDA): branch of the U.S. Government concerned with safety of foods and drugs.

fraction: single treatment dose of radiation; one part of the predetermined total dose.

fracture *(frak'-shur)*: a break in a bone.

- G -

gamma rays *(ga'-muh rayz)*: powerful radiation beams (similar to X-rays) from a radioactive material, such as cobalt; used for radiotherapy.

grade: classification of degree of malignancy of a tumor; in lung cancer, grade I is the least malignant, grade IV is the most malignant.

- H -

hair follicle *(hair fahl'-uh-kul)*: the root of each hair; because the cells are very sensitive to certain types of chemotherapy, temporary hair loss may occur.

- I -

immune system: the bodily system that fights disease.

immunology *(im-yew-nah'-loh-jee)*: study of the body's immune system.

immunotherapy *(im-yew-noh-thair'-uh-pee)*: a treatment for cancer that attempts to stimulate the body's immune system.

implant: a small container of a radioactive substance placed in a tumor, to destroy it gradually.

incision *(in-sih'-zhun)*: a cut through the skin that allows a surgeon to reach underlying tissues and/or organs.

inflammation *(in-fluh-may'-shun)*: reddening and swelling.

infusion *(in-few'-shun)*: process of giving intravenously a medication that has been dissolved in fluid.

intravenous injection *(in-truh-vee'-nus in-jek'-shun)*: a procedure for injecting a liquid substance into a vein, from where it is carried through the bloodstream to all parts of the body.

irradiation *(ih-ray-dee-ay'-shun)*: see radiotherapy.
IV: abbreviation for intravenous injection.

- K -

Krebiozen *(kreh-bi'-oh-zen)*: a substance claimed to be a cancer remedy, but proved ineffective; its use is now illegal.

- L -

Laetrile *(lay'-uh-tril)*: a substance claimed to be a cancer remedy, but proved ineffective; its use is now illegal.
large cell carcinoma: type of lung cancer; cells are large and do not resemble the cells of skin or glands (see epidermoid carcinoma and adenocarcinoma).
larynx *(lair'-inks)*: the voice box, located just above the windpipe.
lead shield: metal plate, through which X-rays cannot pass, used to protect normal tissues from radiation.
lesion *(lee'-zhun)*: an abnormality in an organ or tissue due to disease.
linear accelerator *(lih'-nee-ur ak-sel'-ur-ay-tur)*: type of X-ray machine used to destroy tumor tissue.
lobe: a division of a body organ, such as the lung, marked off by by a fissure on the surface; there are two lobes in the left lung and three lobes in the right lung.
lobectomy *(loh-behk'-toh-mee)*: surgical removal of one lobe of a lung.
lymph nodes *(limf nohdz)*: bean-shaped structures scattered along the lymphatic system; believed to trap germs and other foreign substances to help stop the spread of disease.
lymphosarcoma *(lim-foh-sahr-koh'-muh)*: type of cancer that begins in the lymph nodes.

lymph vessels *(limf vehs'-sulz)*: channels and ducts that drain fluid from the body tissue and carry it to the bloodstream.
lymphatic system *(limf-a'-tik sis'-tum)*: system of lymph vessels and lymph nodes.

- M -

magnetic resonance imaging: diagnostic procedure in which principles of magnetism are used to create pictures of body structures.
malignancy *(muh-lig'-nun-see)*: uncontrolled growth of cells; cancer.
marinate: to soak food with liquids or spices to make them tender and/or more tasty.
Matulane *(mat'-yew-lane)*: trade name for procarbazine.
mediastinoscopy *(mee-dee-uh-sti-nah'-skoh-pee)*: surgical procedure for examining the lymph nodes under the breastbone for the presence of cancer or other disease.
mediastinum *(mee-dee-uh-sti'-num)*: area of the chest behind the breastbone.
medical oncologist: see chemotherapist.
metastases *(muh-ta'-stuh-seez)*: cancer cells that appear in a part of the body other than the site of the initial tumor.
methotrexate *(meth-oh-trex'-ate)*: a chemotherapy drug; may be given intravenously or by mouth.
microscopic *(my-kroh-skah'-pik)*: too small to be seen without a microscope; the microscope is an instrument that uses lenses for making enlarged images of minute objects, such as the cells of the body.
mitomycin *(my-toh-my'-sin)*: a chemotherapy drug; given intravenously; sometimes called mitomycin-C.
modality *(moh-dal'-uh-tee)*: a type or kind of treatment (for example, surgery).

morphine *(mohr'-feen)*: one of the strongest, most effective pain medications.

MRI: see magnetic resonance imaging.

mucus *(mew'-kus)*: a thick liquid produced by the inner lining of the breathing tree; keeps the breathing passages moist and helps trap foreign particles (so they can be carried up and out of the lungs).

Mutamycin *(mew-tuh-my'-sin)*: trade name for mitomycin.

- N -

National Cancer Institute (NCI): a division of the National Institutes of Health (NIH), run by the federal government; works with all aspects of cancer, from basic science research to patient care.

NMR (nuclear magnetic resonance): see magnetic resonance imaging.

- O -

oat cell carcinoma: see small cell carcinoma.

oncologist *(ahn-kah'-loh-jist)*: a physician who specializes in diagnosing and treating cancer.

oncology *(ahn-kah'-loh-jee)*: branch of medicine that deals with the study and treatment of cancer.

Oncovin *(ahn'-koh-vin)*: trade name for vincristine.

- P -

pathologist *(path-ahl'-oh-jist)*: a physician who specializes in the study of normal and diseased body tissues.

petechiae *(pe-teek'-ee-eye)*: tiny reddish or purplish spots caused by the breaking of tiny blood vessels just beneath the skin.
pilot study: experimental use of a treatment in a small group of patients to learn if it will be effective and safe on a broad scale.
platelets: cells in the blood that help blood to clot.
Platinol *(pla'-tin-all)*: trade name for cisplatin.
pleura *(ploor'-uh)*: membrane that covers the lungs and lines the chest cavity.
pleural effusion *(ploor'-uhl ee-few'-zhun)*: fluid that collects between the lungs and the lining of the chest wall.
pleural fluid: see pleural effusion.
pneumonectomy *(new-moh-nek'-toh-mee)*: surgical removal of one lung.
pneumonia *(new-moh'-nee-ah)*: inflammation of a lung.
pollutant *(poh-lew'-tant)*: foreign substance that contaminates the air; usually considered harmful (such as tobacco smoke).
port film: an X-ray picture of the chest made just before radiotherapy, used for correct positioning of the patient.
procarbazine *(proh-kahr'-buh-zeen)*: a chemotherapy drug, given by mouth.
prophylactic *(proh-fil-ak'-tik)*: guarding against or preventing disease.
protocol *(proh'-tuh-call)*: an approved new treatment program still needing study and evaluation, which patients may elect to join.

- R -

radiation physicist *(fiz'-ih-sist)*: a specialist in the use of radiation equipment and calculation of radiation dosage.
radiation therapy: see radiotherapy.
radiologist: a physician specializing in the use of X-rays and similar energy forms for diagnosis and treatment.
radiosensitive: sensitive to the effects of radiotherapy; see radiosensitization.

radiosensitization *(ray-dee-oh-sen-sih-tuh-zay'-shun)*: treatment to make cancer cells more sensitive (and therefore more responsive) to radiotherapy.

radiotherapist *(ray-dee-oh-thair'-uh-pist)*: a physician specializing in radiotherapy.

radiotherapy *(ray-dee-oh-thair'-uh-pee)*: the treatment of disease (such as cancer) by means of X-rays or radioactive substances (such as radium).

radium *(ray'-dee-um)*: radioactive element used in the treatment of cancer.

RBCs: red blood cells; component of blood that carries oxygen to the tissues of the body.

recurrence: return of cancerous growth.

regression: the act of growing smaller or disappearing; used to describe the shrinkage or disappearance of a tumor.

- S -

shielding: use of a device (often made of lead) to protect tissues surrounding a tumor during radiotherapy to the tumor.

simulation films *(sim-yew-lay'-shun)*: X-ray pictures of the chest used for mapping treatment area; taken with the patient in the position to be used for radiation therapy.

side effects: effects of a drug or other treatment that are not desired.

small cell carcinoma: type of lung cancer in which cells are small and round or oat-shaped; also called oat cell carcinoma.

sonogram *(sahn'-oh-gram)*: a picture made by ultrasound equipment to identify cancer in the body.

sputum *(spew'-tum)*: mucus from the bronchial tubes.

sputum cytology *(spew'-tum si-tahl'-uh-jee)*: examination of cells in the sputum, usually used to look for presence of cancer cells.

squamous cell carcinoma: see epidermoid carcinoma.

stress test: a test for measuring heart and lung functions before, during, and after a controlled period of strenuous exercise.

supraclavicular *(sue-pruh-kluh-vik'-you-lur)*: above the collar-bone (clavicle).

- T -

thoracentesis *(thoh-ruh-sen-tee'-sis)*: the removal of fluid, by needle, from the space between the lungs and the chest wall.

thoracoscope: an instrument fitted with a lighting system and telescopic attachment, designed for examining the chest cavity.

thoracoscopy *(thoh-ruh-kah'-skoh-pee)*: surgical procedure in which a thoracoscope is inserted between two ribs in order to examine the chest cavity and the surface of the lung for cancer.

thoracotomy *(thoh-ruh-kah'-tuh-mee)*: surgical procedure in which an incision is made through the chest wall to examine the structures in the chest for the presence of cancer or other disease.

tolerance *(tah'-lur-uns)*: the ability to endure the effects of a drug without exhibiting the usually unfavorable effects.

tomogram *(toh'-moh-gram)*: a series of X-ray pictures that give a three-dimensional view of structures in the body.

toxic: damaging to cells; poisonous.

trachea *(tray'-kee-ah)*: the windpipe; leads from the larynx to the bronchial tubes.

tranquilizer *(tran'-kwil-eye-zer)*: a drug that reduces feelings of anxiety, worry, or fear.

transfer factor: a substance in the blood that may be able to transfer immunity to a certain disease from one person to another.

- U -

ulcerate *(uhl'-sur-ayt)*: to become an open sore; usually accompanied by bleeding.
ultrasound: high-pitched sound waves that can produce a picture of body structures and detect cancer.

- V -

Velban *(vel'-ban)*: trade name for vinblastine.
vinblastine *(vin-blas'-teen)*: a chemotherapy drug, given intravenously.
vincristine *(vin-kris'-teen)*: a chemotherapy drug, given intravenously.
vital organs: refers to the heart, lungs, liver, and kidneys, which are vital to life.
VP-16: trade name for etoposide.

- W -

WBCs: white blood cells; cells that fight infection.

- X -

X-ray machine: term usually used to describe any of several kinds of equipment that give off beams of radiation; see chest X-ray, radiotherapy, cobalt unit, linear accelerator.
X-ray therapy: medical treatment (as of cancer) by controlled application of X-rays.

Index

Questions for My Doctor

Questions for My Doctor

Questions for My Doctor